IVF & Beyond

FOR

DUMMIES®

by Dr Karin Hammarberg

WILEY

Wiley Publishing Australia Pty Ltd

IVF & Beyond For Dummies®

Published by
Wiley Publishing Australia Pty Ltd
42 McDougall Street
Milton, Qld 4064
www.dummies.com

Copyright © 2010 Wiley Publishing Australia Pty Ltd

The moral rights of the author have been asserted.

National Library of Australia
Cataloguing-in-Publication data:

Author:	Hammarberg, Karin.
Title:	IVF & Beyond For Dummies/Karin Hammarberg.
ISBN:	978 1 74216 946 0 (pbk.)
Notes:	Includes index.
Subjects:	Fertilisation in vitro, Human. Infertility — Treatment.
Dewey Number:	618.178059

Cover image: © amlet, 2010. Used under licence from Shutterstock.com

Typeset by diacriTech, Chennai, India

Printed in China by
Printplus Limited

10 9 8 7 6 5 4 3 2 1

About the Author

Karin Hammarberg, RN, BSc, Master of Women's Health, PhD, is an Honorary Fellow at the Melbourne School of Population Health at the University of Melbourne and Deputy Director of the Low Cost IVF Foundation. In 1982 Karin was a member of the team responsible for the first IVF birth in Sweden, and in 1988 she moved to Melbourne, where she became program coordinator for the Reproductive Biology Unit at the Royal Women's Hospital and later also for Melbourne IVF.

During her years of working with infertile couples Karin has initiated and participated in research in a wide range of areas to improve clinical and psychological outcomes for those undergoing IVF. This includes project managing the largest Australian study to date of women's experiences of pregnancy, childbirth and early mothering after assisted conception. She has also collaborated in research about women's reasons for delaying childbearing, men's experience of infertility, couples' decisions regarding frozen embryos, the value of counselling for people considering donor conception, the health and development of IVF-conceived young adults, and the transition to parenthood for first-time mothers at different ages. Karin's research has been widely published in international scientific journals and she's often invited to speak at national and international conferences.

Karin is a member of the Fertility Society of Australia and has served two terms on the Society's Board of Directors. She is also a member of the European Society for Human Reproduction and Embryology (ESHRE) and the Australian Society for Psychosocial Obstetrics and Gynaecology (ASPOG).

Karin is married with two sons and currently lives in Mill Valley, just north of San Francisco.

Dedication

I dedicate this book to infertile couples and individuals who take on the challenges of IVF treatment in their pursuit of parenthood.

Author's Acknowledgements

Over the many years that I've been involved in the areas of infertility and IVF I've had the good fortune of working with, and being mentored by, many extraordinary people. The knowledge and experience I gained from these people has allowed me to write this book and I'm deeply indebted to them. In chronological order they are: Professor Lars Hamberger, who pioneered IVF in Scandinavia; Drs Matts Wikland and Lennart Enk, who established one of the first private IVF clinics in Sweden; the late Ian Johnston, who was the medical director of the team responsible for the first Australian IVF birth and the first Chairman of Melbourne IVF; Dr John McBain, who subsequently became Chairman of Melbourne IVF; Ms Kay Oke, who led the way to make counselling an integral part of IVF; Professor Gordon Baker, who encouraged me to do research; and Associate Professor Jane Fisher at the Key Centre for Women's Health in Society at the University of Melbourne, who was the principal investigator of the study about childbearing after IVF and my PhD supervisor.

I owe special thanks for assistance during the production of this book to Louise Johnson and Tracey Petrillo from the Victorian Assisted Reproductive Treatment Authority for their expert advice on the legal aspects of IVF; Dr John McBain for his technical review; my husband, Alan Trounson, for his help with the chapter about IVF research; Dr Matts Wikland for providing ultrasound images; and Associate Professor Jane Fisher and Dr Heather Rowe for sharing their excellent work on helping new parents through the transition to parenthood.

I thoroughly enjoyed working with the Wiley team. Acquisitions Editor Charlotte Duff saw the need for a resource for people considering IVF and believed I could write it; Bronwyn Duhigg helped me navigate the process of writing a *For Dummies* book; Caroline Hunter was the most wonderful and sensitive editor a writer could wish for; and Gabrielle Packman was a great project leader. I also thank Glenn Lumsden for his illustrations and the US editors for their input.

Lastly, I want to express some personal thanks. My husband, Alan, and our children, Karl and Alex, have given me much-appreciated encouragement and support during the year that I've been glued to my computer; and my 'Wednesday Walkers' friends have listened patiently to accounts of my writing progress — and sometimes lack thereof.

Publisher's Acknowledgements

We're proud of this book; please send us your comments through our online registration form located at http://dummies.custhelp.com.

Some of the people who helped bring this book to market include the following:

Acquisitions, Editorial and Media Development

Project Editor: Caroline Hunter, Burrumundi Pty Ltd

Acquisitions Editors: Bronwyn Duhigg and Charlotte Duff

Editorial Manager: Gabrielle Packman

Production

Graphics: Wiley Art Studio

Cartoons: Glenn Lumsden

Proofreader: Marguerite Thomas

Indexer: Karen Gillen

The author and publisher would like to thank the following copyright holders, organisations and individuals for their permission to reproduce copyright material in this book:

- © Matts Wikland: pages **100, 101** and **102**
- Jane Fisher: page **230** www.whatwerewethinking.org.au

Every effort has been made to trace the ownership of copyright material. Information that will enable the publisher to rectify any error or omission in subsequent editions will be welcome. In such cases, please contact the Permissions Section of John Wiley & Sons Australia, Ltd.

Contents at a Glance

Table of Contents

Introduction

. . . .

*W*hen you're ready to start a family you're full of anticipation about taking on the joys and responsibilities of parenthood. However, if month after month goes by without you falling pregnant, you may get a sinking feeling that something is wrong. Most people take fertility for granted and that's why infertility usually comes as a shock to couples who face it. Having no doubt spent many years trying to *avoid* falling pregnant, it's quite ironic to discover that when you really want a baby you can't conceive. Well, you're not alone — about one in six couples experience fertility difficulties at some time and if, like many of them, you discover that you need IVF to conceive, *IVF & Beyond For Dummies* is your perfect companion.

IVF treatment is like a long and winding detour on the road to parenthood and you may feel a bit dizzy from it all if you do eventually fall pregnant. Drawing from research of women who become mothers after having IVF, *IVF & Beyond For Dummies* also explains how you can deal with the challenges of parenthood.

After 20 years of working as a nurse with infertile couples in IVF clinics and ten years being involved in research about how infertility and infertility treatment can disrupt your life, I've used my combined clinical and research experience to write *IVF & Beyond For Dummies* for those who're contemplating IVF, and their friends and families. If you're 'shopping' for information about IVF, *IVF & Beyond For Dummies* is your one-stop shop. It covers everything you need to know about the medical, technical, emotional, legal and financial aspects of IVF treatment and about life after IVF.

About This Book

To have IVF treatment you need to be equipped with knowledge and patience. Knowledge gives you a heads-up on what IVF treatment entails, makes you feel in control of how you manage your fertility problem and empowers you to make informed decisions along your IVF journey; patience helps you persist with treatment if IVF doesn't work straight away. *IVF & Beyond For Dummies* gives you a comprehensive account of how to prepare yourself for IVF, the steps involved in IVF treatment (including what may go wrong), how infertility and IVF can play havoc with your emotions and test your relationship, and what life after IVF may be like for you.

Whether you're just thinking about having IVF, you're in the middle of treatment or you're on your way to parenthood after IVF, *IVF & Beyond For Dummies* has something for you. The book is a resource for infertile couples, single women and same-sex couples who consider IVF, and those who want to know how they can help a family member or a friend who's in the throes of IVF.

Conventions Used in This Book

To make it easy for you to navigate this book I use some style conventions:

- ✔ Important terms are set in *italics* when they are used for the first time and are closely followed by an easy-to-understand definition. These terms also appear in Appendix B at the end of the book.
- ✔ Sidebars are interesting tangents but not critical to the text.
- ✔ Text preceded by the icons 'Technical stuff' and 'Personal stories' are not essential reading for you to understand the subject at hand, but if you like technical details or enjoy real-life stories, these sections are for you.
- ✔ The field of assisted reproductive technology (ART) is full of abbreviations and acronyms. These are explained within the text and also appear in Appendix A at the end of the book.
- ✔ I have addressed all IVF nurses as 'she', because as far as I'm aware all IVF nurses are female.

Foolish Assumptions

I've made some assumptions about who may find this book useful:

- ✔ Couples who're contemplating IVF
- ✔ Couples who're ready to start IVF treatment
- ✔ People, including singles, who want to know whether IVF is an option for them

- ✔ Couples who've had successful IVF treatment and are looking forward to becoming parents
- ✔ Friends and family who want to find out how they can help someone they care for who needs IVF

How This Book Is Organised

IVF & Beyond For Dummies is divided into seven parts. The first four parts detail the journey from discovering that you can't fall pregnant, to undergoing an infertility investigation to find out why, to having IVF treatment to try to have a family. Part V is the 'beyond' component of the book where I talk about what's special about pregnancy, birth and parenting after IVF. Part VI consists of two lists of useful tips for IVF and beyond; and Part VII contains abbreviations and terms used in IVF, as well as some websites that you may find useful.

Part I: Getting Ready for IVF

Perhaps you've been trying for a baby for many months and nothing has happened. If you think you've waited long enough and want to start doing something to help you conceive, I suggest that you start reading here. In this part, I talk about the steps you can take to find out why you can't conceive and the possible treatment options. I devote a whole chapter to discussing how you may feel when you discover that you're infertile and how to handle the emotional aspects of infertility. I also talk about what you can do to improve your chances of IVF working and how to find an IVF clinic.

Part II: All You Need to Know About IVF

If none of the low-tech infertility treatments work for you, you may consider IVF — the high-tech way of having a baby. In this part, I delve into the legal, financial, medical, technical and — very importantly — emotional aspects of IVF treatment. The more you know about the IVF process and what to expect throughout the stages of IVF, the better you'll manage the stressful nature of the treatment.

Part III: Understanding the Risks of IVF

Australian IVF clinics operate to very high standards and are run by highly qualified professionals who make sure your treatment is safe and efficient. However, like all other medical procedures, IVF treatment is associated with some risks. In this part, I outline the physical and emotional risks of IVF treatment. I also talk about how to move on if IVF doesn't work for you.

Part IV: Pushing the Boundaries

In this part, I describe the IVF add-ons that some couples may need to consider, such as using donor gametes (eggs and sperm) or embryos, using surrogacy or undergoing embryo testing to avoid passing on serious health problems to the child. I also talk about the options of freezing and storing gametes and embryos for future use and look at some of the promising IVF-related research that's going on in the world.

Part V: Beyond IVF

If IVF works for you and you fall pregnant, you and the rest of the world will agree that you've been very lucky! In this part, as you look forward very much to becoming parents, I explain what's special about pregnancy, birth and parenting after IVF. I also share with you some of the experiences of almost 200 IVF mums whom some colleagues and I studied from early in their pregnancies until their babies were eighteen months old.

Part VI: The Part of Tens

The Parts of Tens is a *For Dummies* specialty, providing short, sharp information about areas of interest. In this part, I give you ten tips for surviving IVF and ten tips for new IVF parents. If you read nothing else, the Part of Tens will help you keep sane through the trials and tribulations of IVF treatment and will help prepare you for life as a new parent.

Part VII: Appendixes

As you read this book, perhaps skipping from chapter to chapter, looking at only the parts that interest you, you may come across terms and abbreviations that you don't understand. That's why I include the appendixes. Appendix A spells out the numerous abbreviations that you may come across or hear bandied about and Appendix B provides definitions for these terms and the many others you're likely to encounter on your IVF journey. In Appendix C, you find a list of useful websites.

Icons Used in This Book

To help you get the most out of this book, I include some icons that tell you at a glance whether a section or paragraph has important information of a particular kind.

This icon points you to useful websites.

Over the years that I've been working with infertile couples, I've heard many personal stories that have given me an appreciation of how infertility affects people's lives. I think you'll find some of these stories very pertinent.

This icon points you to important information that you need during your infertility and IVF journey.

If you like to know the nitty-gritty of how things work, this icon directs you to information that's not essential reading but may interest you.

This icon highlights handy hints that can make life easier for you during IVF and beyond.

This icon alerts you to potential problems or difficulties.

Where to Go from Here

You can read this book from cover to cover or use it as a resource that you pull out when you're looking for an answer to a specific question. Depending on where you are on your infertility journey and what particular information you're seeking, you may not need to read everything I have to say — although you're certainly welcome to! Use the Table of Contents to pick and choose the chapters or sections you want to read and skip the parts that deal with matters you've already been through.

Part I
Getting Ready for IVF

Glenn Lumsden

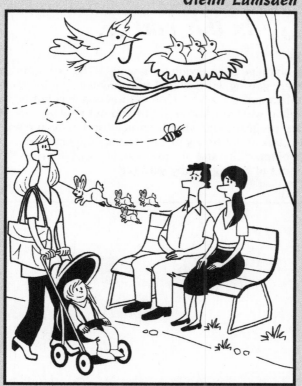

'Since we found out we have a fertility problem, Mother Nature is really giving me the pips.'

In this part ...

So you've been trying for a while to have a baby and are getting worried that you may have an infertility problem and need IVF treatment to conceive. In this part, I explain what you can to do to find out why you aren't falling pregnant and what treatment options you have. I also talk about how you can manage the emotional side of infertility and discuss how you can improve your chances of having a baby with IVF.

Chapter 1

Taking First Things First

*L*ike the majority of couples, you may have found that deciding to start a family is a major relationship commitment that takes time. But having made the decision and stopped contraception, you probably felt excited and full of expectations about this next stage of your life. Most couples take fertility for granted and don't expect to have trouble getting pregnant. Yet 10 to 15 per cent of couples trying for a baby fail to fall pregnant in the first 12 months. Month after month passes without any sign of pregnancy and frustration sets in. If you're in this situation, now's the time to take the bull by the horns and acknowledge that you may have a fertility problem.

In this chapter, I provide some tips about finding an infertility specialist and explain the tests you're likely to undergo to find out why you haven't conceived. I also describe some of the simpler types of infertility treatment that your doctor may suggest you try before you move on to in-vitro fertilisation (IVF) treatment.

Becoming a parent is a life-changing experience that throws you into a spin of emotions. If you have to put a lot of effort into having a family, you feel very lucky when you finally have a baby. But caring for a new baby is one of the hardest jobs around and having IVF doesn't make the job any easier or less demanding. So I also introduce you to some of the common misconceptions (pardon the pun!) about parenting after IVF.

Finding Out Why You Don't Get Pregnant

As soon as you suspect that you have a fertility problem, you need to confirm your suspicions and find out what sort of problem you have, because this determines your treatment. Some detective work is needed here and you may have to see several doctors before you discover the cause of your infertility.

A fertility problem is a challenge that you and your partner should tackle together. Whenever possible, make sure that you can both attend the required medical appointments.

Don't waste precious time doing nothing. Your chances of having a baby, with or without IVF, depend a great deal on the female partner's age (I give you statistics about this in Chapter 3). So, if you've been trying unsuccessfully for a year or more, don't get talked into waiting just a little longer — especially if you're aged in your mid-thirties or above.

Talking to your family doctor

Your family doctor is usually the first person you turn to with your concerns. Expect your doctor to

- Confirm that you're aware of the optimum time of the month for conceiving
- Order some basic tests to confirm that the female partner ovulates (releases an egg) regularly and the male partner produces sperm
- Take a detailed medical history and an even more detailed reproductive and sexual history of you and your partner
- Undertake a physical examination of you and your partner

Assuming everything seems okay, your doctor may suggest that you wait a bit longer before consulting an infertility specialist.

However, if the tests your family doctor recommends don't explain why you haven't conceived, or they reveal a problem that requires treatment, you need to move to the next level of care. You need a referral from your family doctor to see a specialist and most doctors are only too happy to provide a referral for infertility issues.

Finding an infertility specialist

There are several types of specialist that you may see for an infertility problem:

- ✔ *Andrologists* are specialists in matters relating to the male reproductive organs.

- ✔ *Gynaecologists* specialise in matters relating to the female reproductive organs.

- ✔ *Infertility specialists* are gynaecologists who specialise in the treatment of infertility. If such a specialist practises in the area where you live, ask your family doctor for a referral straight to the top!

If you live in an urban area, you may have several infertility specialists to choose from. Rather than your family doctor simply referring you to one particular specialist, you may want to think about what's important to you and ask to be referred to the specialist who best fits your preferences in terms of the following issues:

- ✔ **Distance to travel:** You're likely to need to see the infertility specialist a number of times, so not travelling too far may be an important consideration.

- ✔ **Doctor's gender:** Do you prefer a female doctor or a male doctor?

- ✔ **IVF expertise:** Not all gynaecologists perform IVF, so if you think you may need IVF ask about this *before* choosing a specialist.

- ✔ **IVF treatment location:** Infertility specialists sometimes practise in different locations, but they perform IVF at one particular clinic. Knowing which clinic a specialist uses may help you to make your choice.

- ✔ **Recommendation:** If you know someone who's had infertility treatment, it may be worth asking that person to recommend a specialist.

- ✔ **Waiting time:** Some specialists have long waiting lists for new patients — if you have to wait months for an initial appointment, you may consider seeing someone else.

If you live in a rural area or small town, you may not have access to an infertility specialist, but any gynaecologist who practises nearby can undertake your infertility investigation.

Busting the myth that stress causes infertility

Well-meaning (or maybe not so well-meaning) friends and relatives may suggest that you can't fall pregnant because the female partner (it's always the female partner) is too stressed or too focused on her career. It sounds tempting to think that stress may be the reason for your inability to conceive and some women take this message on board.

The theory that being too stressed can stop you from getting pregnant has been the subject of much research and to my knowledge there's no good evidence to support this theory. In fact, it's very unhelpful to suggest to someone that stress causes infertility because — guess what — if you're infertile and believe that it's because you're too stressed, this makes you feel even more stressed! However, plenty of research shows that infertility itself is a very stressful experience. How stressful depends on the individual, but an unfulfilled wish for a child is inevitably distressing.

So don't get caught up in the idea that you somehow cause yourself to be infertile just because you're too stressed, work too much or want a career. Disregard 'friendly' advice to take a holiday, cut your hours at work or avoid going for a promotion: Such action isn't going to increase your chances of having a baby, and it may cause you to miss out on career opportunities.

You must be happy with how you and your infertility specialist get along because you're at the mercy of this doctor throughout your infertility investigation and treatment. Bedside manners matter, so if you're not comfortable with a specialist, consider looking for someone who better fits your needs.

Having the infertility investigation

After you've found a suitable infertility specialist, the specialist has to determine the cause of your infertility in order to decide what type of treatment you may need. Many different types of tests and investigations are available and you start with the simplest and least invasive, moving onto the more-complex tests until a cause is pinpointed.

The infertility investigation often takes quite some time and effort, and you can easily find yourself getting a bit impatient because all you want to do is to get treated. Try to keep your cool because getting the right diagnosis prevents you from going down the wrong treatment track — saving you valuable time and money.

Testing him

The main test for the male partner is usually a sperm test or semen analysis, which is analysed in a specialist laboratory. You receive detailed instructions about ejaculating into a special jar (very clinical) at home and where to deliver the sample. The World Health Organization (WHO) standards for what's considered normal in a sperm sample are accepted by most infertility clinics. The lab report details several things about the sperm, including the following:

- **Antisperm antibodies:** These can cause clumping of sperm, rendering them unable to move and fertilise the egg. A normal sperm sample has no sperm antibodies.

- **Concentration:** The number of sperm per millilitre of ejaculate. WHO standard: more than 20 million per millilitre.

- **Count:** The total number of sperm in the ejaculate. WHO standard: 40 million or more.

- **Morphology:** The percentage of sperm that have normal shape. WHO standard: more than 15 per cent.

- **Motility:** The percentage of sperm that move forward vigorously. WHO standard: 50 per cent or more.

- **pH:** Should be alkaline.

- **Volume:** The amount of ejaculate expressed in millilitres. WHO standard: 2–5 millilitres.

- **White blood cell count:** There should be very few white blood cells; a lot of white blood cells can be a sign of an infection.

Each component of the report reveals something about your fertility but the components need to be considered together to make sense. From the analysis the specialist can tell you whether the quality of your sperm may be a reason why you haven't conceived. If your sperm test is normal, you probably won't be tested further. However, if your sperm test reveals severe abnormalities, the specialist may ask you to undergo a testicular biopsy, during which tiny pieces of testicular tissue are taken via a needle and examined under the microscope to see whether you're producing sperm. Depending on the outcome of the biopsy, you may need a blood test to check your hormone levels and to get a final diagnosis regarding your sperm.

Tongue twisters

The terms that are used to describe different sperm problems deserve a mention, because they sound like extremely weird creatures indeed!

- **Asthenospermia:** Not enough sperm swimming forward

- **Azoospermia:** No sperm

- **Oligospermia:** Fewer sperm than normal

- **Teratospermia:** Too many sperm with abnormal shape

If you have several sperm problems, these weird words are put together to create even stranger words!

- **Asthenoteratospermia:** Not enough sperm swimming forward and too many with abnormal shape

- **Oligoasthenoteratospermia:** Too few sperm, too many with abnormal shape and not enough swimming forward

- **Oligoteratospermia:** Too few sperm and too many with abnormal shape

Testing her

The female partner may need to undergo several tests and procedures. These tests check whether you have an ovulatory problem and whether your ovaries (where the eggs are stored), fallopian tubes (which transport the eggs to the uterus) and uterus are normal.

- **Checking ovulation:** A common reason why couples have trouble conceiving is that the woman rarely or never ovulates. During ovulation, the woman's body releases a mature egg that if fertilised by a sperm grows into a baby. Two hormones regulate ovulation and the menstrual cycle:

  - Follicle-stimulating hormone (FSH)

  - Luteinising hormone (LH)

These hormones are produced by a small gland in the brain called the pituitary gland and they interact with two other hormones, oestrogen and progesterone, which are produced by the ovaries.

To check whether you ovulate, you may have blood tests to measure these hormones and most likely also a vaginal ultrasound examination, where your ovaries can be seen on a screen.

Around ovulation time your body temperature increases slightly. In the 'bad old days', a woman with a suspected infertility problem would be asked to take her temperature every morning before getting out of bed, sometimes for months on end. The doctor used these measurements to work out if and when the woman was ovulating. Don't get talked into following this procedure — blood tests and ultrasound are much more reliable (and far less time-consuming) ways of verifying ovulation.

✔ **Looking at your fallopian tubes:** If ovulation isn't the problem, the next test examines whether your fallopian tubes are healthy. A vaginal ultrasound examination gives some information about the fallopian tubes but a laparoscopy is more exact. A *laparoscopy* is an internal abdominal examination, for which you're given a general anaesthetic. The doctor makes a small incision close to your navel through which an instrument is inserted so that the doctor can thoroughly examine the organs in your pelvis, including your fallopian tubes and uterus. This examination may reveal that the reason you don't conceive is due to a tubal problem (I discuss this issue in the section 'Female causes' later in the chapter), but may also show that everything looks just the way it should.

✔ **Peeking into your uterus:** To make sure that the uterine cavity — the inside of the uterus — has all that it takes to provide a 'good home' for a pregnancy, you may undergo one or both of the following tests:

✔ **Hysterosalpingogram (HSG):** Contrast (which works like a dye) is injected into your uterus via the cervix (the neck of the womb). Your uterus and fallopian tubes are then X-rayed in order to check the outline of the uterine cavity and whether fluid flows freely from your uterus through the fallopian tubes.

✔ **Hysteroscopy:** A thin telescope-like instrument is inserted into your uterus through your cervix to check that no lumps and bumps are distorting the uterine cavity (the inside of the uterus). During the procedure your doctor also takes small samples of the endometrium (the lining in the uterus). The endometrium changes in response to the hormonal changes that occur during the menstrual cycle and the samples are tested to make sure that your endometrium has the right appearance.

Getting a diagnosis

After all the testing has been completed and the results have been reviewed, the specialist can give you the verdict. There may be one or several reasons why you can't conceive. Roughly speaking, one-third of infertility cases are due to male factors, one-third are due to female factors and one-third are caused by a mixture of male and female factors or have no apparent cause. Depending on the cause, the specialist then outlines your treatment options.

Male causes

The male partner may have various problems with his sperm, ranging from relatively minor problems such as a slightly reduced sperm count to major problems such as no sperm at all in the ejaculate. If no sperm appear in the ejaculate, a testicular biopsy can reveal whether this is because sperm aren't being produced or whether a blockage is stopping the sperm from mixing with the ejaculate. Sperm problems may also be caused by hormonal deficiencies.

Female causes

While male infertility revolves around a sperm problem, female infertility can result from a variety of problems with hormones, ovulation, the fallopian tubes or uterus. And as if that wasn't enough, fertility declines with the female partner's age. Here's a snapshot of the most common causes of female infertility:

- **Ovulation troubles:** The most common cause of female infertility is a problem with ovulation. *Amenorrhea,* the complete absence of periods and *oligomenorrhea*, infrequent and irregular periods, mean that ovulation doesn't happen at all (*anovulation*) or happens very infrequently.

  Ovaries contain follicles in various stages of development. *Follicles* are fluid-filled little cysts where eggs grow and mature before ovulating. Between 10 and 20 per cent of women have polycystic ovaries, an excess number of tiny follicles in their ovaries, and ovulate very infrequently; and some 5 per cent of women suffer from a more severe condition, polycystic ovarian syndrome — a hormone imbalance that affects many bodily functions, including ovulation.

- **Tubal blockages:** Another major cause of infertility is damaged fallopian tubes. One or both tubes may be completely or partially blocked, which sometimes causes them to fill up with fluid (so-called *hydrosalpinx*). Some tubes can become immobilised by adhesions — scar tissue that 'glues' them to other tissue when they should be moving freely. And if you've had an *ectopic pregnancy* (a pregnancy that grows in a fallopian tube rather than in the uterus), you may have had one or other fallopian tubes surgically removed.

- **Uterine problems:** *Uterine fibroids* are benign tumours of muscle and other tissue that grow on the surface, inside or within the walls of the uterus. The fibroids vary in size; the bigger they are, the more havoc they can cause. About 40 per cent of women aged 35 and older have one or more fibroids. While fibroids don't always cause infertility, they can distort the uterine cavity and make it difficult for a pregnancy to grow.

- ✔ **Endometriosis is trouble all over:** *Endometriosis* is a condition whereby the tissue that lines the inside of the uterus finds its way to other places in the body such as the ovaries, fallopian tubes and outer surfaces of the uterus, bowel and bladder. These colonies of endometrial tissue react in the same way as the endometrium in the uterus to the hormone changes that occur during the menstrual cycle, so that in effect you get 'internal periods'. It's difficult to know how common endometriosis is because many women have the condition unknowingly and conceive without trouble. For others, however, endometriosis is a debilitating condition that causes chronic pelvic pain, problems relating to the bowel and bladder, bleeding and infertility.

- ✔ **Having too many birthdays:** Fertility declines naturally with age, so sadly just adding years to your life decreases your chance of having a baby. I explain the gloomy statistics for how age affects fertility in Chapter 3.

A bit of both

Some couples share everything, including their fertility problem. At the end of your infertility investigation, you may be told that your sperm is a bit dodgy, you have a bit of endometriosis and your fallopian tubes don't look too flash! If you have several causes for your infertility, the specialist will probably refer you straight to IVF treatment.

Unexplained causes

For some 10 to 15 per cent of couples, their infertility tests come back normal: There's no apparent reason why they can't conceive. *Idiopathic* or unexplained infertility can be very frustrating and many couples with idiopathic infertility say that not knowing *why* they're infertile makes things even worse.

Scientists believe that many cases of idiopathic infertility have genetic, molecular or immunological origins but the tests to prove this haven't yet been invented.

Dealing with Your Feelings

Even if you *suspect* that you have a fertility problem, receiving the actual diagnosis of infertility suddenly makes it all real and scary. This isn't how you planned it! Books written about the emotional impact of a diagnosis of infertility compare it's magnitude with the devastation of other major life events such as the loss of a loved one or divorce.

You have no way of knowing how long your infertility will last. You may fall pregnant next month or you may never conceive. This uncertainly is one of the most difficult things about being infertile: Limbo isn't a good place to be.

Unfortunately, you need to face the fact that it may take you a lot of time, effort and money to reach your goal of parenthood and that getting there will consume a great deal of emotional energy. The best way to handle this is to acknowledge and try to understand your own and your partner's feelings and reactions and to find ways of dealing with negative feelings such as worry, sadness and hopelessness so that these feelings don't take over your life completely. I devote the whole of Chapter 2 to this topic and hope that it helps you on your infertility journey.

Dealing with the stress and strains of infertility is a major challenge and if you add to that the emotional ups and downs of IVF treatment, you can be forgiven for feeling under the pump from time to time. I discuss how you can prepare for the emotional roller-coaster ride of IVF treatment in Chapter 9; and in Chapter 11, I cover what's known about the short- and long-term risks of infertility and IVF to your mental health and wellbeing.

Getting Ready for Action

Knowing that you need some type of infertility treatment doesn't necessarily mean that you're ready for it. You may need some time to get over the shock of the diagnosis and gather some well-needed energy to embark on treatment. On the other hand, you may be eager to get going with treatment and feel better knowing that you're actively doing something to have the baby you long for.

Here are some things you need to do before undergoing treatment, whether you decide to wait or start straight away:

- ✔ **Confirm that you're both ready for infertility treatment:** Infertility treatment is tough on you, so you and you partner must *both* be ready to take it on. One partner dragging the other to the clinic doesn't work and often ends in tears. If you disagree about when to start treatment, try working out a compromise because you'll need each other's support when you're in the throes of treatment. In Chapter 2 I talk about the importance of the two of you working together like a well-oiled team on this.

- ✔ **Consider how much time and money you'll need:** If you need IVF treatment, this will consume a lot of time, physical and emotional energy, and money. The physical and emotional energy drain is difficult to prepare for — you just have to be ready for it and deal with it when it happens. But knowing that you need to attend the clinic several times during each treatment cycle can help you plan ahead to reduce the risk of work/treatment clashes (and the stress that this causes). I talk more about juggling your job and treatment in Chapter 3. And even though Australians are very fortunate compared to many others in terms of how IVF is funded by Medicare and private health insurance, you'll still have considerable out-of-pocket expenses when you undergo treatment. If you have plenty of money that may not be a problem, but if not you'll have to budget for treatment. I talk about the financial aspects of IVF treatment in Chapter 3.

✔ **Look after your health:** Research shows very convincingly that certain lifestyle factors influence the chances of infertility treatment working. All the usual stuff about following a healthy diet, not smoking and not drinking too much alcohol applies, but you can do other things to improve your odds too, such as losing weight if you need to and exercising regularly. You find more information about how to optimise your chances of having a baby (and improving your general health) in Chapter 3.

Possible Low-tech Alternatives

For some types of infertility problems — for example, if your fallopian tubes are totally blocked or you have a severe male factor problem — the only way you can conceive is through IVF. However, some causes of infertility can potentially be fixed with less invasive and less costly types of treatment. You don't need a shotgun to kill a fly, so as a general rule you start with the simpler forms of treatment, if they're an option considering the cause of your infertility, before moving onto IVF if you don't get pregnant.

Stimulating egg production

Ovulation induction may be an option for you if the only problem you have is that you don't ovulate regularly. Sometimes, a course of clomiphene citrate (CC), a synthetic anti-oestrogen, is all that you need to fall pregnant. You take CC in tablet form for five days, starting during your period. The drug 'tricks' the pituitary into thinking that your levels of oestrogen are low. In response, the pituitary starts to produce more follicle-stimulating hormone (FSH), which — and there are no points for guessing this — stimulates the growth of follicles in your ovaries.

Using ultrasound, your doctor then checks your ovaries' response to the drug. The ideal response is one to two growing follicles, and when these are about to ovulate you need to be ready for sex! If you have no response your dose of CC can be increased. However, some women are CC-resistant so no matter what dose they take, their ovaries don't respond.

If you don't respond to CC your doctor may suggest that you take a course of FSH injections to stimulate ovulation. You will need to be monitored carefully to ensure that you don't produce too many follicles, however, because that puts you at risk of having a multiple pregnancy.

Timing ovulation

Another way to optimise conditions if you have idiopathic infertility or ovulation problems is to time your ovulation so that you can have sex at the time when conception is most likely to happen. Whether you ovulate spontaneously or with tablets or injections, knowing when ovulation happens helps you to step up your efforts at the right time. To pinpoint exactly when you'll next ovulate (to within a few hours), your doctor gives you a single injection of human chorion gonadotrophin (hCG) when the follicle size as measured with an ultrasound examination indicates that the egg is ready. Having sex in the subsequent two to three days is your best chance to get pregnant.

Helping the sperm to meet the egg

You can try artificial insemination homologue (AIH) (insemination with your partner's sperm) if you have idiopathic infertility or a very minor male factor problem. To make sure that eggs and sperm are given the best possible opportunity to meet and greet (and hopefully get together), the sperm are inseminated into your uterus just before ovulation (which is timed using hCG, as explained in the section 'Timing ovulation'). Your partner needs to supply a sperm sample, of course, which the lab staff prepare, and then the doctor or nurse deposits a small amount of concentrated sperm solution at the top of your vagina or in your uterus. Hopefully, nature then takes care of the rest.

If you have a severe male factor problem and decide to use donor sperm (discussed in Chapter 13), you have the same procedure but it's called artificial insemination donor (AID) or donor insemination (DI).

If you have a severe male factor problem and female-related fertility problems, you need IVF with donor sperm.

When all else fails — next stop, IVF

After several unsuccessful attempts with one or a combination of ovulation induction, timed ovulation and artificial insemination homologue/donor, it's time to bring in the big guns: IVF.

Don't spend too many months on 'low-tech' treatments because the older you get, the more your chance of getting pregnant declines, even with IVF. As a result, you need to get to the most effective treatment for you without delay.

Moving On to IVF: The High-tech Way to Get Pregnant

Whether you've already tried other forms of infertility treatment or are told that IVF is the only way for you to have a baby, making the decision to start IVF treatment is a big one. Nonetheless, many couples at this stage also feel a sense of relief that they're finally going to be actively doing something that gives them a chance of having a family.

To help make your decision, you need to find out as much as you can about IVF before you start treatment. This includes what the law says about who can have IVF, what happens in an IVF cycle, what your chances are of the treatment working and what the risks of treatment are.

Who can have IVF in Australia?

There are laws and regulations governing IVF in many Australian states relating to who can access IVF treatment, what kinds of records clinics need to keep, what clinics need to do to make sure that couples can make an informed decision, how long eggs/sperm/embryos can be frozen, the rules for donation of eggs/sperm/embryos and other matters.

These laws and regulations change from time to time and vary between the states. For example, in the past only legally married heterosexual couples were able to access IVF in some states, but today married and de facto couples can access IVF in all states and in some states same-sex couples and single women are also eligible for IVF. In addition, some states require identifying information about egg/sperm/embryo donors and recipients to be kept in central registers so that when donor-conceived children grow up they can find out who their genetic parents are, while in other states such information-keeping is up to the individual clinics.

I explain the legal and regulatory aspects of IVF in Chapter 4 and in Chapter 13 I outline the laws and regulations governing donor conception.

Jumping the hurdles of IVF

You come across a range of health-care professionals on your way through IVF treatment and in Chapter 4 I introduce you to the many members of your IVF team. It's very important that you feel you receive the best possible care, so I also discuss how you can ensure that the members of your IVF team respond to your needs — and what you can do if they don't.

IVF is like a set of hurdles that you have to jump in order to get to the finishing line — hopefully with a baby in your arms! In Chapter 5 I describe the obstacle course, what it takes to get over those hurdles and what may go wrong along the way.

IVF is often likened to an emotional roller-coaster ride. In Chapter 9 I explain how the ups and downs you go through during an IVF treatment cycle can throw you off course and how you can get back on track again.

If you're interested in technical details, I explain the actions and possible side effects of the drugs you take for IVF in Chapter 6, what happens in the IVF lab in Chapter 7 and how you can estimate your chances of having a baby with IVF in Chapter 8.

Knowing the risks

As with all things high-tech, IVF involves some risks that you should know about before starting treatment. In Chapter 10 I explain the physical risks during the treatment cycle itself as well as the treatment-related risks to you and your baby during pregnancy and after the birth. IVF is high-stress as well as high-tech, and you can expect to feel pretty anxious and sad from time to time. Much research has been carried out into how infertility and IVF treatment can affect your emotional wellbeing and I talk about the take-home messages from this research in Chapter 11.

One of the biggest risks of IVF is that treatment doesn't work. Sadly, sometimes the much-wanted pregnancy doesn't eventuate, or is lost. In Chapter 12 I discuss these scenarios and ways to move on with your life if IVF doesn't work for you.

IVF-plus

More complex forms of treatment have evolved from the 'original' IVF treatment, some of which you may need in your quest to start a family:

- ✔ **Third-party reproduction:** Today, some 10 per cent of IVF treatment cycles involve using donor gametes (eggs and sperm) or embryos to have a baby. The big question that arises in such cases is whether a child born as a result of the donation should be able to find out who the donor is. I discuss the arguments for and against in Chapter 13.

- ✔ **Use of a surrogate:** Less common than using donor material, but perhaps more controversial, is the use of a surrogate to carry the pregnancy and give birth. If the female partner doesn't have a uterus or is unable to carry a pregnancy, the embryo can be transferred to another woman's uterus. After the birth the baby is given to the infertile couple, who raise the child. I explore the complex issues involved with surrogacy in Chapter 14.

- ✔ **Freezing sperm and embryos:** Freezing techniques have come a long way and there are now very efficient ways of preserving sperm and embryos. Eggs can also be frozen, but this has proven more difficult and less successful. In Chapter 15 I discuss gamete and embryo freezing and some of the tricky decisions you sometimes have to make when you have frozen embryos.

- ✔ **Pre-implantation genetic diagnosis:** We all carry good and not so good genes but some of the really bad genes can cause severe conditions such as haemophilia and cystic fibrosis. If you know that members of your family suffer from an inheritable life-threatening condition, you can check whether the genes that cause the condition are present in an embryo before it's transferred. This technique, known as pre-implantation genetic diagnosis, can help you to have a healthy child if you're at risk of passing on a genetic disease. I explain the ins and outs of this very high-tech process in Chapter 16.

Beyond IVF

An IVF pregnancy is a happy ending to a very trying time. But it's also the beginning of a new journey into the unknown. After you put the worries about getting pregnant behind you, you find that you start to worry about the pregnancy, the birth and the welfare of your baby. Of course, couples who conceive without IVF also have such worries, but new research shows that some aspects of pregnancy, childbirth and parenting are a bit different and perhaps more complex after assisted conception.

In Chapter 18 I explain how you may be feeling during your pregnancy and how you can prepare for the birth and in Chapter 19 I talk about the big event of the birth.

Caring for a new baby is one of the most wonderful but also the most difficult tasks in life. In Chapter 20 I offer some advice to make the transition to parenthood a bit easier and let you in on some of the tricks of the trade of new parenthood. And in Chapter 21 I talk about how life slowly gets back to normal after the first few crazy months of new parenthood.

Chapter 2

Why Us? Going Through the Emotions of Being Infertile

*B*y the time you're ready to have children you've probably spent a good part of your life trying to *avoid* getting pregnant. In today's world couples can very easily 'turn off' their fertility by using contraception, and of course they expect that something that can be 'turned off' can also be 'turned on' again. The realisation that you've spent all this time turning off something that didn't even work often comes as a great surprise. Most people take their fertility for granted and think of being fertile as 'normal', which can make you feel 'abnormal' if you're infertile — not easy to take on the chin!

Being diagnosed as infertile is a big blow if parenting is part of your life plan. As with any other major life crisis, the diagnosis stirs up a lot of emotions that can be very difficult to handle. Most couples describe stages of shock, denial, anger, sadness and worry about whether they'll ever have a baby.

In this chapter, I discuss some common reactions to a diagnosis of infertility. By understanding how and why infertility plays havoc with your emotions you should find dealing with your feelings is easier and you can look for ways to avoid your emotions taking over your life completely. In addition, I outline different sources of support that can be useful throughout the infertility journey.

Reacting to Your Infertility Diagnosis

Even if you've long suspected that you have an infertility problem, the actual diagnosis of infertility can come as a shock. Like many people, your initial reaction to the news may be disbelief: 'There must be a mistake here! Maybe the test results are wrong, or they've been mixed up?' After it all sinks in you may feel angry: 'Why us? What have we done to deserve this? This is so unfair!' You may also feel guilty, blaming your infertility on something you did in the past: 'It's probably because I had that termination when I was 16', 'If only I'd been more careful when I went backpacking 20 years ago I wouldn't have been infected with *Chlamydia*!' Over time, you may also experience all or some of the following:

✔ A sense of being overwhelmed

✔ Feelings of isolation, because infertility can be difficult to talk about

✔ Sadness and grief about not being able to do what's 'only natural'

✔ Worry about whether you'll ever have a baby

Rest assured that such reactions are normal: There's no right or wrong way to respond to such life-changing news.

Dealing with shame and guilt

You may also feel shame about not being able to accomplish something that you and everyone else expects of you, or about your sexual capacity being questioned. And you may feel guilty if, for a fleeting moment, you wish that your best friend would miscarry or you resent your sister's new baby.

Shame and guilt aren't useful emotions: They only make you feel worse. Try to keep these emotions out of your repertoire, but if they do creep up on you, confront them and do your best to shake them off. Remember:

✔ Don't be too hard on yourself for not being able to feel ecstatic with joy when your best friend announces that she's pregnant.

✔ You've done nothing to 'deserve' being infertile.

Counting your losses

Your reactions to your (hopefully temporary) loss of fertility are really responses to a whole raft of losses, including loss of:

- A dream, because you always planned to have children
- Control, as you can't do what others seem to do so easily
- Identity, because you always imagined being a parent one day
- Genetic continuation in the family tree, which may be short of a limb if you can't have children
- Social inclusion with all your friends and family who have children

If you've had the misfortune of experiencing pregnancy loss, the struggle to get pregnant again is a constant reminder of the baby or babies you almost had. Grieving for the loss of an unborn child is hard because society doesn't usually have rituals for acknowledging this kind of bereavement. People don't always know how to talk about pregnancy loss or how to show their support for couples who've lost a pregnancy. Added to this, you may not have told anyone about your pregnancy and with no funeral to express your feelings, dealing with your loss can be a very lonely experience.

Talking about infertility and pregnancy loss can be difficult but those close to you may find it easier to be supportive and caring if they know how you really feel. So don't hold back about your feelings and pretend you're fine when you're not. Love and acknowledgement of your grief can make you feel much better: Give your loved ones a chance to show their support.

In Chapter 11, I talk about coping with pregnancy loss after IVF treatment and give you some tips on working your way through the grieving process.

But everyone else can have a baby!

When you've been trying unsuccessfully to get pregnant, you see babies everywhere. Suddenly, everyone in your orbit has a baby and none of them appears to have had any trouble getting pregnant. It all seems grossly unfair and can make you feel sad and left out. Some women who're able to have kids at the drop of a hat can appear unconcerned whether they have another child or not. How fair is that? Of course, you know that these things have nothing to do with your infertility, but they can still make you feel angry.

How she may feel

For many women, motherhood is the ultimate expression of femininity and so you may feel less of a woman if you can't have children. In fact, you may feel less of a person altogether and it's not uncommon that the infertility experience dints your self-esteem and self-confidence, hopefully not in a lasting way. I talk about ways to maintain your self-confidence in Chapter 11.

You're certain to feel sad and worried about the future ('Will I ever have a baby?') and you may also wonder if your relationship with your partner will survive or crumble under the pressure of it all.

How he may feel

We used to think that men with an infertility problem feel vulnerable and weak because the infertility reduces their masculinity. Although this may have been true in the past, recent research shows that most men today don't equate fertility with masculinity, so this stereotype no longer holds.

In fact, infertile men see fatherhood as a highly valued and important life goal. Childlessness is no less distressing for them than for their partners. So feelings of loss, sadness and worry are all normal.

Challenging research

In a study conducted in Australia, 112 men who'd been diagnosed as infertile five years previously filled out questionnaires about what had happened in terms of their infertility since they were diagnosed. Almost all of them (96 per cent) had gone through some form of infertility treatment with their partner and most had become fathers (87 per cent), either as a result of the treatment or after conceiving spontaneously or adopting a child. The men were asked to indicate whether they agreed with a number of statements about parenthood, and their responses, shown at right, challenge the stereotypes that men believe that fertility is linked to masculinity and that having children is less important for men than for women.

- Parenthood is as important to me as to my partner (84 per cent)

- Having children makes a marriage a family (70 per cent)

- The disappointment of not having children is greater for the woman than for the man (42 per cent)

- Having children makes a stronger bond between husband and wife (71 per cent)

- A man can never be sure of his masculinity until he is a father (10 per cent)

- Becoming a mother makes a woman truly female (15 per cent)

Avoiding the blame game

Wanting to pin the blame on someone or something when you're facing difficulties in life is normal. That someone or something becomes the target of your frustration and gives you an outlet for your negative feelings. But if an infertility problem lies with just one partner, blame can cause havoc in the relationship. A fertile man may resent not being able to have children because his partner has blocked tubes, and a fertile woman may wish she'd married someone with a normal sperm count.

Infertility is not 'his problem' or 'her problem': It's a couple problem that you have to deal with together, so avoid the blame game.

The burden of being the partner with the fertility problem can affect the dynamics of a relationship too. The infertile partner may become withdrawn and feel inferior because she or he is 'causing the problem', and may even offer to end the relationship so that the fertile partner can find someone else to have a family with. This then places pressure on the fertile partner to bend over backwards to be reassuring and understanding. Talking openly about your feelings is the best way to avoid damaging your relationship.

Dealing with Other People's Reactions

As if dealing with your own feelings about being infertile isn't enough, you're also confronted with other people's feelings and opinions about your infertility. Being prepared and thinking about how to best handle other people's reactions can help limit the impact of their lack of understanding of infertility.

Talking about infertility: How, and to whom?

Like many others, you may feel that infertility is a very private matter and want to keep it to yourself and your partner. Unfortunately, not talking about the issue can make things more difficult for you, because you're on your own when life is really tough and some support from others would be really helpful.

Although you obviously don't want to tell the whole world about your fertility problems, if you tell people you feel close to, you'll most likely find that they're only too keen to be there for you and help in any way they can.

Putting up with nosy family and friends

Some people are good at putting their foot in it and frequently they're the ones closest to you. Your mother or mother-in-law may be impatient for grandchildren, putting her foot in it when she asks: 'And when are you two going to stop thinking about yourselves and start having a family?' The best man at your wedding may put his foot in it when he says 'About time you got her pregnant, mate' (nudge-nudge, wink-wink). And your best friend may put her foot in it when she says 'Now that I'm pregnant, why don't you have a baby too, so we can do this together?' (as if you weren't already trying!).

People spout such insensitive and intrusive comments without realising that they can be very hurtful. Unless you're prepared to explain all about your pregnancy difficulties, perhaps you can get them to pull their heads in by saying something like 'Well, these things don't always happen easily' or 'We'll let you know just as soon as it happens'.

Trying for a second (or third) baby

If you already have a child or children and are trying for a second or (goodness me!) third or fourth child, people are often less sympathetic for some reason. They may say things like 'You should be grateful for what you have' (as if you weren't) or 'Don't be greedy' (if you weren't having trouble conceiving, no-one would suggest that wanting more than one child is greedy).

Dealing with *secondary infertility*, when you already have a child or children and have trouble conceiving again, can be as difficult as coping with *primary infertility*, when you experience difficulty having your first child. Don't believe those who say that you don't have the same right to try for a second or third child as for a first child.

Starting over with a new partner

If you and/or your partner have children from a previous relationship and want a child together but discover that you can't, others may think that this situation isn't such a big deal since you already have children in your lives. But you experience the same sense of loss and sadness at not being able to extend your family as if you didn't already have children.

Some reasons for wanting children are perceived as more worthy than others and some are perceived as downright 'selfish', such as you and your partner each having three children from previous relationships but wanting a child together. Yet most reasons for wanting children are 'selfish' — people have children to fulfil their own wishes and life goals, and no reason is more or less worthy than others.

Working As a Team

I can't stress too often that infertility has to be treated as a *couple problem*, irrespective of who has the bit that 'doesn't work'. If you're going to survive IVF, you really need to do everything you can to work together and try to support each other through the treatment, especially when things don't go to plan.

Research shows that couples who have IVF have better-than-average relationships: Probably a bit of self-selection is going on here. Only couples who have a strong commitment to each other and a strong desire to have children choose to have IVF. But relationships are tested on the infertility journey and you need to keep reminding yourself to look out and care for each other while you battle on.

Being on the same page

One of the tricky things about dealing with the emotional side of infertility is that each partner may be in a different phase of working out what to do. For example, your partner may be keen to start treatment, whereas you still feel angry and haven't yet reached a more constructive phase. Your different personalities can also make you handle the difficulties in different ways. One of you may want to forget all about the problem and hope that it goes away, while the other faces up to the problem and starts to look for ways to solve it.

If you and your partner aren't 'on the same page', try to find a way to move forward that works for you both. To do this you need to understand each other's position and find some middle ground. Be open with each other, be honest about your feelings and be willing to listen to your partner's point of view.

Treating yourself and each other kindly

When you're struggling with infertility, you can easily lose sight of the fun side of life. Suddenly, everything is overshadowed by your unfulfilled wish for a child. The infertility journey can be long, so you can't afford to let it consume you totally and rob you of all the pleasures in life.

Try to keep doing the things that you enjoy doing, be it sport, reading, going to the movies or escaping somewhere for the weekend. More than ever you need the energy and sense of wellbeing that these kinds of activities provide. Be kind to yourself and to your partner, spoil each other and indulge whenever you can in anything that makes you feel good.

Having sex on demand; where did the fun go?

Infertile couples commonly feel that the joy and pleasure they used to experience in their sexual relationship goes out the window when the focus is on baby making rather than on love making. Trying hard to time sex at the most fertile stage can be the biggest turn-off and can dampen your enjoyment. It may even give him 'performance anxiety' and cause erection difficulties. And her libido may take a beating from tension about infertility and doubt about ever falling pregnant.

Even if your sex life isn't as pleasurable as it used to be, don't forget to give each other plenty of affection and physical closeness. Going away for the weekend and deciding not to take your infertility problems with you gives you a break and may bring on lust and the urge to have sex just because you love each other!

Finding Support

You may be doing everything in your power to keep on an even keel in the stormy waters of infertility, but still feel as though you may sink when the next big wave comes your way. You get no points for battling on alone and can improve your chances of surviving the storm by grabbing hold of one of the life-saving devices that are around. One or all of the following sources of support may help save you.

Talking things over with a buddy

Talking to your partner about how you feel is all well and good, but if you're both hurting badly, your partner can't give you all the support you need. Having someone outside your relationship to confide in — someone you trust and feel can provide ongoing support — may be immensely helpful. A good buddy is happy to lend you a shoulder to cry on. Perhaps this person may be your mum, or your sister, or your best pal from work. Set aside time to meet up with your buddy and give vent to your feelings. Opening up may be hard at first, but after you've broached the subject the going usually gets easier.

Wanting to talk about how you feel, especially when you're facing difficulties, is perhaps more common among women than men. But women and men can both benefit from leaning on a kind and sympathetic friend or relative in the testing times of infertility.

Discovering help online

Endless opportunities exist to connect online with people anywhere in the world with whom you share experiences, and infertility experiences are no exception. Hundreds of websites and chat rooms are dedicated to couples with fertility difficulties. You can access these virtual support groups from your desk at home. The groups can be very useful as a sounding board and for making you realise that you're not on your own.

If you find talking about infertility or your feelings difficult, internet-based support may be more suitable for you; you can stay anonymous and such interaction may be less confronting than sharing your feelings with someone close to you.

Two good places to start are

- ACCESS, Australia's National Infertility Network (www.access.org.au)
- Australian Infertility Support Group (www.nor.com.au/community/aisg)

I list some other useful websites to visit in Appendix C.

Some websites provide infertility-related medical information and advice. The quality of this information varies considerably: Treat all such information with caution. By all means, use the internet to become more knowledgeable about infertility and its causes and treatments, but don't treat the information you find as gospel. Each couple's circumstances are different and unique and you need individualised advice, which only those familiar with your detailed medical history can provide.

Joining a support group

Support groups are groups of people who get together because they share a problem, usually a medical condition. Members of infertility support groups give each other moral support and understanding. Joining such a group helps you realise that you're not the only couple in the world struggling to have a family. Most local support groups are associated with particular IVF clinics or are devoted to a particular type of infertility. You can find contact details for all IVF clinics in Australia and New Zealand on the Australian Infertility Support Group's website (www.nor.com.au/community/aisg). I list the largest support groups in Appendix C.

Calling in the professionals

If all else fails, or you feel that talking to an expert in the field of the psychological and social consequences of infertility would be beneficial, your best bet may be to see an infertility counsellor or psychologist.

Counselling services are an integral part of all Australian IVF clinics and couples are encouraged to use these services whenever they need to — before, during or after infertility treatment. Counsellors provide useful information, individual or couple support, relationship counselling and generally help you to stay sane during the course of infertility. I talk more about the role of counsellors in IVF in Chapter 4.

If you're not yet part of an infertility clinic, you may not be able to access clinic counselling services. But you can still contact your local clinic and ask for the name of an independent psychologist or counsellor with an interest in infertility issues.

Chapter 3

Setting the Perfect Scene

In This Chapter

▶ Getting into shape for pregnancy

▶ Understanding the facts about ageing and fertility

▶ Finding the right clinic for you

▶ Coping with treatment charges

▶ Juggling your job and IVF

*I*VF treatment gives millions of couples the opportunity to become parents, but unfortunately the treatment doesn't work for everyone. IVF has an element of 'luck of the draw' and you can't do much about that. However, you can do several things to improve your chances of success before you start treatment.

In this chapter, I explain how certain lifestyle factors influence the outcome of IVF and what you can do to improve the odds in your favour. I also outline how to find the IVF clinic that best suits your needs and what you can do to reduce your out-of-pocket expenses for IVF treatment.

Improving Your Chances of IVF Success

The success rate for IVF treatment has greatly improved since the late 1970s when the technique was first introduced. Although your chance of having a baby with IVF depends largely on factors beyond your control — such as how many eggs you produce in response to your drug protocol and whether your eggs and sperm turn into healthy embryos — recent research shows that getting into shape *before* starting IVF treatment can influence the odds in your favour. This mostly involves things you should be doing anyway to stay healthy — there's no rocket science to it!

Stopping smoking

No two ways about it: Smoking is *bad* for your health. If you smoke and are trying to fall pregnant, consider these facts:

- ✔ **Smokers have lower fertility than non-smokers:** The many toxic substances in tobacco smoke have negative effects on sperm count, follicle development, ovulation, transport of the egg through the fallopian tubes, fertilisation and embryo development — yes, pretty much every aspect of fertility!

- ✔ **Smoking reduces your chances of IVF success:**

  - Women who smoke need nearly twice as many IVF cycles to conceive as non-smokers.

  - The male partner smoking decreases IVF success rates.

  - The risk of early pregnancy loss after IVF treatment is *twice* as high for women who smoke as for non-smokers.

  - Passive smoking reduces the chance of IVF pregnancy by *20 per cent*.

Quitting smoking can be extremely difficult, because nicotine is a very addictive substance, but if you and/or your partner smoke, make a pact to kick the habit before you start IVF treatment.

Many effective methods are available to make quitting smoking easier. To find out how you can help yourself to stop smoking once and for all:

- ✔ Call the Quitline on **13 18 48**

- ✔ Talk to your family doctor

- ✔ Visit the Australian government's Quit Now website at `www.quitnow.info.au`

Counting your drinks

Here's some sobering (pardon the pun) news about how alcohol affects pregnancy. Studies show that alcohol:

- ✔ Decreases fertility

- ✔ Increases the risk of miscarriage

- ✔ Negatively affects the unborn child, particularly in the first few weeks after conception

The evidence about the effects of alcohol consumption on IVF success is not as clear cut as for smoking, but one study found that women who drink alcohol produce fewer eggs, have a lower chance of pregnancy and face a higher risk of miscarriage than women who don't drink. If the male partner drinks, this also increases the risk of miscarriage.

Researchers are yet to determine exactly how much alcohol you need to drink to run these risks. However, to be on the safe side, try to avoid alcohol, or at least drink very little, while you're trying for a baby.

Cutting back on caffeine

Caffeine is a stimulant that many people consume by drinking coffee, tea or certain types of soft drink. Researchers have discovered that women who consume a lot of caffeine — more than three cups of coffee per day — may take longer to conceive.

Not much is known about the effects of caffeine on IVF outcomes, but one study found that the higher a woman's caffeine intake, the lower her chances of a live birth. At this stage, men's caffeine consumption hasn't been found to affect IVF success.

You can continue to enjoy the odd latte while you're on IVF treatment, but if you consume several caffeine beverages per day, cutting down on your intake is a good idea.

Reducing stress

Some researchers believe that psychological stress — like feeling worried, sad, overwhelmed or unable to enjoy things — can have a negative effect on a woman's reproductive capacity, but no solid evidence exists to prove that this is the case. Perhaps feeling down can dampen your desire for sex and decrease the frequency of intercourse, which naturally reduces your chances of conception.

The effect of psychological stress on IVF outcomes is also ambiguous. When IVF doesn't work for a couple, both partners naturally feel sad and worried about whether they'll ever be able to have a child — so a connection definitely exists between negative IVF outcomes and psychological stress. But whether this stress then decreases the chance of the couple's next IVF treatment working isn't clear. I talk more about the cause–effect relationship between infertility and psychological stress in Chapter 1.

Regardless of whether feeling positive and optimistic improves your chances of IVF success, when you feel upbeat your life is more enjoyable. So, for this reason alone you need to look after your emotional health, and I discuss some of the ways in which you can do this in Chapter 2.

Psychological stress is a normal response to infertility and infertility treatment, so don't bash yourself up if you don't feel positive and optimistic all the time. And, if IVF treatment doesn't work for you, please don't blame yourself.

Watching your weight

Your *body mass index (BMI)* gives an indication of the amount of body fat you have and is calculated from your weight and height. A normal BMI is in the range from 18.5 to 25.

If you and/or your partner have a BMI lower or higher than this, it can cause hormonal imbalances that disrupt ovulation and reduce sperm quality, which in turn decrease the likelihood of conception. In addition, obesity increases a woman's risk of miscarriage, pregnancy complications and needing a Caesarean section delivery.

Studies of the relationship between a woman's weight and her chances of having a baby with IVF show that obesity almost *halves* the probability of pregnancy.

If you're carrying a lot of excess weight you're most likely painfully aware of just how difficult losing weight can be. You may have tried any number of methods and found that none of them work in the long run. The problem with most diets is that they're difficult to stick to because they're very prescriptive or exclude too many food items.

Calculating your BMI

To calculate your BMI, first obtain your height in metres (m) and your weight in kilograms (kg). Then complete the following calculation:

For example, if you're 1.7 m tall and weigh 65 kg, your BMI is 65 ÷ 2.89 (1.7 × 1.7) = 22.5 — in the normal range.

$$BMI = weight\ (kg) \div height^2\ (m^2)$$

Consider instead a holistic approach to weight management geared towards lifestyle modifications in a supported environment. Many fertility clinics offer *lifestyle modification programs* so that overweight couples who're contemplating IVF can lose weight before starting treatment. Typically, these programs run for three to six months and involve weekly attendance in a group setting. A range of health-care professionals provide you with diet advice, exercise regimes, support and information about ways to improve your physical and emotional health, as well as your chance of pregnancy.

You don't need to lose a lot of weight to see positive effects, so don't be disheartened if you have a lot of weight to lose. Dropping five to ten kilograms helps establish ovulation, improves the chance of IVF working and reduces your risk of miscarriage and other pregnancy complications — and, of course, improves your general health too.

Eating well

A well-balanced diet provides all the nutrients you need without too many calories and is essential not only for your health in general but also for the wellbeing of a growing foetus. So, to be sure that your diet is as good as can be, take a good look at what you eat and make any necessary adjustments *before* you get pregnant.

Lifestyle modification programs

Lifestyle modification programs were pioneered in Adelaide by Dr Anne Clark and her colleagues in the 1990s. In one of their studies, 87 women who had a BMI over 30 and were infertile — most of them because they didn't ovulate — attended a weekly program for six months. This program included exercise, education about food and diet, and emotional support. Although the women on average lost only a modest amount of weight (6.5 kg), after six months most were ovulating spontaneously. Of the 67 women who completed the program,

78 per cent became pregnant and 67 per cent had a baby. The women who didn't get pregnant smoked, attended less than two-thirds of the classes or still had a BMI over 40 at the end of the program.

Similar programs are now available at numerous IVF clinics throughout the country and are an increasingly popular low-tech alternative for couples trying to improve their chance of having a baby.

A healthy diet involves no magic and I'm sure that you know what that diet is — the tricky part is sticking to it! Just in case you need a reminder, the food pyramid in Figure 3-1 shows the composition of a healthy diet. Make sure that the bulk of your daily diet consists of items at the bottom of the pyramid, like cereals, pasta and rice; munch on three to five servings of veges and two to four servings of fruit; have two to three servings each of low-fat dairy products and meat/poultry/fish/beans for protein; and go *very sparingly* on the sweet goodies and fats at the top of the pyramid.

If you follow a healthy diet you won't need to take any vitamins or other supplements, except folic acid (see the section 'Taking folic acid'). However, if you have trouble eating all the right things every day, you can take a multivitamin that has the right amount of vitamins you need.

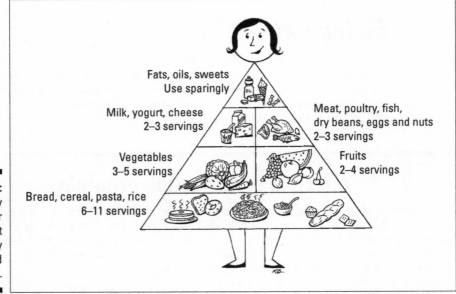

Figure 3-1:
A shapely reminder about what to eat every day — and how much.

Taking folic acid

Folic acid is essential for healthy cell growth and reproduction. Evidence abounds that getting enough folic acid before conception and during the early stages of pregnancy greatly reduces the risk of the baby having neural tube defects such as spina bifida.

So where can you find folic acid? Foods like leafy green vegetables, fruits, dried beans, peas, wholegrain cereals and nuts are rich in folic acid, but the best option when you're planning to fall pregnant is a daily supplement, which you can buy over the counter at any chemist shop.

Getting on your bike

Being physically fit benefits your general health as it helps you to fend off nasties like heart disease, high blood pressure, diabetes and osteoporosis. Regular exercise and a healthy diet are the cornerstones for maintaining good health and optimising physical and emotional wellbeing.

Making time for physical activity is important, but when you're trying to get pregnant you mustn't overdo things: Marathons and other extreme sports are out for now, as they can adversely affect ovulation.

Weighing up complementary therapies

More and more people are looking to alternative or complementary therapies to optimise their health. Couples who want to have a baby are no exception and those who're infertile are often keen to try anything that may help them conceive.

Many of the available therapies are geared towards improving general wellbeing and emotional health. Massage therapies, reflexology, yoga, meditation, stress management, relaxation and aromatherapy are all ways to help you handle the stresses of life and many infertile couples find these forms of therapies helpful.

Think carefully, though, about using ingestible therapies like naturopathy, homeopathy and Chinese herbal treatments, which involve taking substances for specific conditions. The effects of most herbal therapies haven't been tested in the way that society expects prescription medication to be tested and little is known about their safety, benefits and potential side effects. Many people believe that anything herbal is good for their health — or at least not bad for it. However, often the herbs used to improve fertility are quite potent and they can interfere with the fertility drugs that your doctor prescribes.

If you're undergoing infertility treatment, you *must* discuss any herbal treatments you take with your doctor to make sure that the herbs don't mess up your treatment. For example, the following herbs used to enhance fertility may be harmful during IVF treatment:

- ✔ **Black cohosh and red clover:** May increase oestrogen levels.
- ✔ **Dong quai:** Has a blood-thinning effect.
- ✔ **Mugwort and feverfew:** May be harmful to the unborn baby.
- ✔ **Red raspberry leaves:** Can cause uterine contractions.

Avoid these six herbs at all costs.

Beating the Clock: Age Counts, So Get Started!

Most people know that a woman's chance of having a baby decreases with age, but few are sure at what age this starts to happen. Many also believe that men's reproductive capacity is unaffected by age — just look at Charlie Chaplin fathering children into his seventies!

The reality is that fertility declines with age for both women and men: For women, the sad fact is that fertility starts to decline from about age 25. In addition, as you get older, the risk of having a child with birth defects increases.

In this section I share some of the realities concerning the impact of age on natural fertility and on your chances of success with IVF.

- ✔ If you're over 35 years of age and thinking about starting IVF, the information won't be terribly helpful to you: The best you can do is to get started as soon as you can.
- ✔ If you're in your late twenties or early thirties and hoping to finish your house renovations, save some more money or advance your career before you start IVF, the information may save you disappointment down the track.

Age and fertility

A baby girl is born with her lifetime's supply of eggs. As she ages, so do her eggs. Theoretically reproduction is possible from *menarche* (the first period she has) until *menopause* (when her periods stop). But her chance of having a baby drops 3 to 5 per cent per year after she reaches the age of 30 and the rate of decline is even faster after she hits 40.

In addition, older eggs are more likely to be chromosomally abnormal, and this has two important effects:

✔ The risk of miscarriage increases, because most miscarriages occur due to the foetus not having the right number of chromosomes

✔ The risk of the baby having chromosomal abnormalities such as Down syndrome increases

The link between women's age and fertility has been known for a long time, but a relatively recent discovery is that partners of older men take longer to conceive than partners of younger men.

Age and IVF success

A common misconception (no pun intended!) is that IVF can help you have a baby if you put off starting a family until later in life. After all, movie stars seem to have no problems having babies in their forties. Well, in many cases these women use eggs donated by younger women to conceive, although such a fact isn't usually publicised. (I cover donor conception in Chapter 13.)

Age is one of *the most important factors* in determining your chance of having a baby with IVF. In Chapter 8 I show you exactly how age affects your IVF treatment, but the long and the short of it is that your odds of having a successful pregnancy decrease dramatically as you approach age 40.

Data from Australia and New Zealand show that:

✔ The average age of women who have IVF is 35 years.

✔ Women under the age of 30 have a 26 per cent chance of having a baby after one IVF cycle.

✔ Women over the age of 40 have only a 6 per cent chance of having a baby after one IVF cycle.

Taken together, the best advice if you're contemplating IVF is to get started *now*.

Reasons for delaying childbearing

In a study at a Melbourne-based IVF clinic, 152 women aged over 35 who were about to start IVF treatment completed a survey about their reasons for delaying childbearing. The women's average age was 38.9 years and the mean length of their current relationship was 7.5 years. From a list of ten reasons they were asked to endorse all those that applied to them. The five most commonly stated reasons for delaying childbearing were

✔ I wanted children earlier but I was not in a relationship. (50 per cent)

✔ We wanted to be financially secure before having a family. (32 per cent)

✔ I haven't been interested in having children until recently. (26 per cent)

✔ I wanted to pursue my career before having a family. (19 per cent)

✔ I was unaware that my chance of having children is age-related. (18 per cent)

Not having a partner is obviously a reason beyond personal control, but the women who gave this reason had been in their current relationship for five years on average. Lack of awareness of the impact of age on fertility may have contributed to the other common reasons for delaying childbearing.

The take-home message here is that if you meet your partner later in life and you want to have children, don't wait too long; and if you're approaching 35 and your life ambitions include having a family, put baby making at the top of the list!

Choosing an IVF Clinic

About 75 clinics around Australia provide IVF services. Your family doctor or the doctor looking after your infertility investigation may routinely refer his or her patients to a particular clinic, but you may prefer to choose the clinic yourself.

If you live in a city you may have several IVF clinics within a ten-kilometre radius of your home or workplace. So how do you know which clinic's right for you? Researching the clinics helps you make an informed decision. Start by gathering as much information as you can.

If you live in a rural or semi-rural area, you may have only one clinic within a reasonable distance (and even that may be a long way away!) so you may not be able to contemplate going anywhere else. Follow the suggestions in this section to find out as much as you can about that facility, so that you're as well-prepared as possible before you start treatment.

Checking out your local clinics

The best starting point for your research is the *Fertility Society of Australia (FSA)*. This organisation represents doctors, scientists, counsellors, nurses and consumers in reproductive medicine. FSA's Reproductive Technology Accreditation Committee (RTAC) monitors clinics around the country to make sure that they provide services according to industry standards. IVF clinics can operate only if they pass the auditing process and are granted a licence by RTAC.

The FSA's website (www.fsa.au.com) has a section listing the names and locations of all IVF clinics in the country. Click on the RTAC tab at the top of the page and then on Accredited Units: The clinics appear, sorted by states. Use this information to find the clinics in your local area and then visit the websites of the clinics that interest you to check out what each clinic has to say about its services. Clinic websites are often very glossy and full of promises but they also contain useful information. By comparing the contents of several clinics' websites you get a feel for how the clinics operate and what services they provide.

Sometimes you can't find all the information you need online. Don't hesitate to phone any of the clinics you're interested in to find out more. Also ask whether they send out information packs to prospective clients — for example, some clinics have educational DVDs outlining what treatment involves.

In addition, you may want to ask each clinic how treatment information is provided and who explains what the procedures involve. Before you can give informed consent to treatment you need to get your head around a lot of information, such as the downsides to treatment and the potential side effects of drugs. So you need to be sure that the clinic explains this information clearly to you.

Narrowing down your choices

After you've tracked down your local clinics and assessed the services they offer, you may find that one clinic appeals more than the others. Or you may still be undecided. Either way, before you make your final decision ensure that you consider the following specific issues:

- **One-stop shops:** Most clinics are one-stop shops, so that you complete your whole treatment cycle under the one roof. This means that you go to the one place for all your blood tests, ultrasound examinations, egg collection, embryo transfer and appointments with doctors, nurses and counsellors. However, at some smaller clinics you may need to travel to different locations to get everything done. If you have the option, you may prefer a one-stop shop.

✔ **Success rates:** The ultimate success of IVF treatment and its related procedures is the birth of a healthy baby at term. The facts and figures about clinics' success rates at IVF treatment can be difficult to follow because clinics don't always measure the same things.

For example, Australian statistics show that if 100 women start a stimulated IVF cycle (treatment with hormone injections to stimulate egg production) approximately:

- 90 have eggs collected

- 80 have embryos available for transfer

- 25 have a positive pregnancy test

- 20 give birth

Using these statistics, a clinic that quotes its success rate as the number of pregnancies (including those that later miscarry) per embryo transfer gives its success rate as 31 per cent (25 ÷ 80), whereas a clinic that measures its success as the number of live births per started treatment cycle gives the figure as 20 per cent (20 ÷ 100) — quite a big difference for the same end result. When you compare clinics you need to make sure that you compare like with like.

I discuss how to get a realistic picture of your own chance of having a baby, considering your circumstances, in Chapter 8.

✔ **Travel to and from the clinic:** You'll make many trips to the IVF clinic over the course of your treatment, so you need to consider travelling time to the clinic, transport options and parking facilities. If you don't drive or have access to a car, then the clinic that's serviced by public transport may be best for you. If time is important to you, find out which clinic is easiest to get to.

✔ **Treatment options:** Large clinics usually provide a full range of treatments but smaller clinics may be limited in the services they offer. Treatments that may not be available in smaller clinics include

- *Blastocyst transfer*, whereby embryos are cultured for up to five days before being transferred to the uterus (see Chapter 7)

- Egg freezing (see Chapter 15)

- *Pre-implantation genetic diagnosis (PGD)*, whereby embryos are genetically tested before they are transferred (see Chapter 16)

- Treatments involving donor eggs, sperm or embryos (see Chapter 13)

> ✔ Some large clinics have smaller satellite clinics spread out geographically for the convenience of their clients. If you attend a satellite clinic that doesn't offer a type of treatment you need, chances are you can have that part of the treatment at the large main clinic.

Covering the Costs of Treatment

Australia is one of the few countries in the world where the health-care system covers a substantial proportion of the financial costs of IVF treatment and where women aren't limited in the number of treatments they can have. As a result, an Australian couple may pay ten times less than an American couple for an IVF cycle.

Each clinic sets its own fees and you can find out the exact total cost of your treatment from the clinic's accounts department. In addition to the clinic fees you may need to pay for hospital admission for egg collection and for anaesthetist fees. Also expect to have considerable out-of-pocket expenses, which vary depending on the clinic you attend and the type of treatment you need. For example, the cost quoted for a treatment cycle doesn't include the costs of certain drugs that you're prescribed.

Make sure that you get an estimate of *all* treatment-related costs *before* you start, so that you don't get any nasty surprises.

Medicare cover

Tax payers using IVF see their taxes at work! A large proportion of the costs of IVF treatment are covered by Medicare. Currently, if your out-of-hospital medical expenses, including IVF, exceed $1,126.00 in one calendar year you're eligible for the *Extended Medicare Safety Net* (EMSN), under which Medicare covers 80 per cent of any additional out-of-hospital costs in that calendar year. However, Medicare sets an upper limit on the benefits that can be paid under the EMSN for IVF services.

Medicare rules are revised from time to time, so although this is true at the time of writing, check with your clinic's accounts department for the latest updates.

You need to register for the Extended Medicare Safety Net in order to claim its benefits. Registration involves filling in the appropriate form. You can download this form at www.medicareaustralia.gov.au and register directly online, or you can register at your local Medicare office. To find your local office call **13 20 11**.

After you start treatment, the clinic provides you with statements of the various charges you pay, which you take to Medicare for partial reimbursement.

To enjoy Medicare benefits you need a current referral from your family doctor to your infertility specialist. Referrals to specialists are valid only for one year, so keep an eye on the date of your referral and ask your doctor to renew the referral before it expires.

In addition to Medicare cover, under the government's Pharmaceutical Benefits Scheme certain drugs used in IVF are provided free of charge to patients (see Chapter 6 for more information). This is a blessing, because the drugs used to stimulate the ovaries are very expensive.

Private health insurance

Private health insurance helps you with the costs associated with in-hospital treatment for IVF, such as for egg collection, as well as pregnancy and childbirth-related costs you incur as an in-patient. Insurance companies vary in the length of time they want you to be a member before you can claim reimbursement for IVF-related expenses. They also vary in what they reimburse and how much, so if you don't already have private health cover, make sure that you check these conditions carefully before signing up.

Making Treatment Work with Work

You're likely to experience frustrating time clashes between your IVF treatment and work commitments. During your course of IVF treatment you attend the clinic for appointments with doctors and nurses and for blood tests, ultrasound examinations, egg collection and embryo transfer. Some of these visits are scheduled well in advance, allowing you to plan ahead and reduce the disruption to your work. But sometimes you have to visit the clinic at short notice or at an inconvenient time work-wise, which adds to the stress of treatment.

If you tell your employer that you need time off work to attend appointments for IVF treatment, you may well find that your employer is sympathetic and keen to accommodate the necessary interruptions. In such cases, disruptions can be minimised.

However, you may not want people at work knowing that you're having infertility treatment. You can try making up excuses for your late arrivals and disappearances during the working day, but you won't find too many plausible excuses and sooner or later your boss or work colleagues may start to grizzle about your absences.

If you don't want work to know about your IVF treatment, ask your doctor for a medical certificate to give to work to cover your absences and tell your boss that you have medical appointments.

Part II
All You Need to Know About IVF

Glenn Lumsden

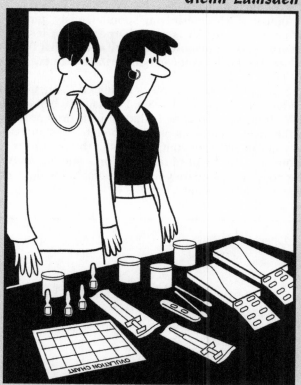

'Remember when the only equipment we needed was candlelight and soft music?'

In this part ...

Compared with conceiving spontaneously, getting pregnant with IVF is much harder and far less pleasurable. But the more you know about what IVF involves, the better you can handle the treatment cycles.

In this part, I outline how IVF is regulated in Australia and introduce you to your IVF team. I explain each stage of the IVF treatment process, including your drug protocol and the magic that takes place in the lab. I also advise how you can estimate your chances of the treatment working for you. Finally, I take you for a ride on the IVF roller-coaster to prepare you for the emotional ups and downs of IVF treatment.

Chapter 4

The Law and the Team

*I*n Australia, IVF services are highly regulated and IVF clinics are scrutinised to ensure that they meet the clinical and scientific standards set out in the Reproductive Technology Accreditation Committee (RTAC) professional code of practice. In addition, various pieces of legislation stipulate who can access IVF and what clinics can and can't do. In this chapter, I give you an overview of the laws, regulations and guidelines that govern IVF.

I also introduce you to all the people you meet from the clinic when you undergo IVF treatment. IVF is a team effort — but you're the most significant member of the team. Always keep in mind that your needs are important and that you have every right to expect the rest of the team to make your time on the IVF program as smooth-running as it can be. You should be well-informed about everything that happens during your treatment, able to access staff when you need them and clear about the full costs of your treatment. In this chapter I explain how to get the most out of your IVF team and ensure that communication runs effectively.

Legally Speaking: Understanding How IVF Services Are Regulated

In Australia, assisted reproductive technologies such as IVF are heavily regulated by federal and state government legislation as well as professional bodies. Overall, such regulation is beneficial for couples seeking IVF treatment because you can be sure that clinics have high standards of care.

All IVF programs have to abide by the following rules and regulations:

- ✔ *Research Involving Human Embryos Act 2002* (Cwlth) and *Prohibition of Human Cloning for Reproduction Act 2002* (Cwlth), both of which regulate research involving embryos.

- ✔ The National Health and Medical Research Council (NHMRC) *Ethical Guidelines on the Use of Assisted Reproductive Technology in Clinical Practice and Research 2004*, which cover the ethical side of providing IVF services.

- ✔ The Fertility Society of Australia's Reproductive Technology Accreditation Committee (RTAC) Code of Practice for Assisted Reproductive Technology Units, which describes in detail how clinics should be run. The RTAC audits IVF clinics every year to make sure that clinics offer the highest possible standards of care. Only clinics that meet the terms of the code are certified.

Accessing IVF treatment

Various state laws cover who can access IVF, what you need to do before having IVF treatment and what happens when couples or individuals use donor sperm, eggs or embryos (see Chapter 13 for more detailed information on this process). All states and territories allow heterosexual married or de facto couples to access IVF treatment (although in South Australia you have to have lived together for at least five years to qualify!), but the situation isn't as clear cut for single women and homosexual couples.

State IVF laws

The following states have their own laws regulating IVF clinics:

- ✔ **New South Wales:** The Assisted Reproductive Technology Regulation 2009 under the *Assisted Reproductive Technology Act 2007* (NSW) ·

- ✔ **South Australia and Northern Territory:** *Reproductive Technology (Clinical Practices) Act* 1988 (SA)

- ✔ **Victoria:** *Assisted Reproductive Treatment Act* 2008 (Vic.)

- ✔ **Western Australia:** *Human Reproductive Technology Act* 1991 (WA)

Single women and homosexual couples

For single women and lesbian couples the rules for accessing IVF vary between the states. Some states distinguish between medical and social infertility and allow single women and lesbian couples who can't have babies because of a medical problem to access IVF, but don't allow access to women who don't have or don't want a male partner. *Reproductive tourism* is a term coined to describe women who cross state borders to access reproductive services that they can't get in their home state.

The long and the short of the state rules for accessing IVF for single women and lesbian couples are as follows:

- **New South Wales, Western Australia and Victoria:** Single women and lesbian couples can access IVF, irrespective of whether they're medically or socially infertile.

- **Queensland, Tasmania and the Australian Capital Territory:** Individual IVF clinics decide whether to treat single women and lesbian couples.

- **South Australia and Northern Territory:** Single women and lesbian couples can access IVF only if they're medically infertile or are at risk of passing on a serious genetic condition. (I explain how IVF is used to avoid passing on 'bad' genes in Chapter 16.)

Successful legal challenges

The following successful legal challenges to the old South Australian and Victorian laws that stopped single women from accessing IVF have gone some way to improving single women's access to infertility treatment in those two states:

- In 1996 Gail Pearce, a single women, claimed that the *South Australian Reproductive Technology Act* discriminated against single women on the basis of their marital status. The Supreme Court agreed and since then in South Australia single women can access IVF (provided they're medically infertile or at risk of passing on a severe genetic disease).

- In 2000 Dr John McBain took the case of his patient, Lisa Meldrum, to court and was successful in arguing that the *Victorian Infertility Treatment Act* contradicted the federal *Sex Discrimination Act*. The court ruled that in Victoria single women who are medically infertile or at risk of passing on a severe genetic disease could access IVF. Since then Victorian laws have become even more inclusive, and now socially infertile single women and lesbian couples can also access infertility services.

With the exception of Victoria, state laws are silent on gay male couples but a number of gay couples have entered into *surrogacy* agreements with women outside Australia and brought their babies back to Australia to be raised. (I explain more about surrogacy in Chapter 14.)

Legal prerequisites

New South Wales, Queensland, Tasmania, Western Australia and the Australian Capital Territory have no legal prerequisites for accessing IVF but in South Australia, the Northern Territory and Victoria you can't access IVF if:

- ✔ You've been convicted of a sexual or violent offence
- ✔ You've lost custody of a child

In addition, in all states and territories clinics must give you plenty of verbal and written information explaining the ins and outs of treatment before you start and you have to sign a bundle of consent forms (I talk more about this in Chapter 5). I once heard that you sign more consent forms for IVF treatment than for a heart transplant! Victorian couples are even more informed: They're required by law to meet with an infertility counsellor before embarking on IVF treatment. (I discuss the benefits of counselling in Chapter 5.)

Using donor material

Some couples need to use donated eggs, sperm or embryos to have a baby. This is called *donor conception* and I explain the processes involved in Chapter 13.

When donor sperm was first used some 40 years ago to inseminate a woman whose partner was infertile, the common wisdom was that the procedure was best kept secret and no-one — including a child born as a result of the treatment — should be told that donor sperm was used. Today, attitudes have changed: Most people believe a child has the right to know his or her genetic origin and so more and more countries are introducing legislation to allow young adults to find out information about the donor.

In Australia laws concerning donor conception vary between the states and territories. I outline the main points of difference in Chapter 13.

Working With Your IVF Team

Entering the world of IVF, you find a great number of people ready to attend to you. IVF is a team effort, and you're the most significant member of the team. Your needs are important: You should be kept informed about your treatment and staff should be available to answer your questions when you need them.

Introducing the team members

Your IVF team members are highly skilled professionals and in this section I explain the different roles they play. Each person has a particular job to do and each and every one of the IVF team is crucial to your journey through the IVF process.

Don't forget to include yourself as part of the IVF team: You're an expert — on yourself! You're as important as any other team member. So ensure you actively involve yourself in the treatment process: Ask plenty of questions if you're not sure about something, consider carefully the options presented to you, make informed decisions and take charge of the things you *can* control.

Infertility specialist

Infertility specialists are doctors who've spent many years training in obstetrics and gynaecology with the Royal Australian and New Zealand College of Obstetricians and Gynaecologists (RANZCOG). After they qualify these specialists become Fellows of the College and can add the very impressive string of letters 'FRANZCOG' after their name. Some take on even more study and have a formal qualification in the subspecialty of reproductive endocrinology and infertility (CREI), which allows them to add 'CREI' to their credentials.

You're either assigned an infertility specialist (your 'IVF doctor') when you first visit the clinic or your family doctor refers you to an IVF doctor (see Chapter 1) who's responsible for your care throughout the whole IVF process. To begin with, he or she orders tests and investigations in order to pinpoint the reason why you can't fall pregnant (I discuss the infertility investigation in Chapter 1). Then, using this information and considering your age and reproductive history, your IVF doctor engineers a treatment plan that's tailored to your particular circumstances. He or she discusses this plan with you, explains the steps involved and gives you an estimate of the chance of the treatment working for you.

Assuming you're happy with the plan and go ahead, your IVF doctor then follows your progress during each IVF cycle you undertake, directing other team members to manage your treatment (I describe the steps involved in a cycle in Chapter 5). At some clinics your IVF doctor performs all the procedures, but at other clinics a number of IVF doctors work together as a team and you may or may not see your own doctor on the day you have a procedure. But, rest assured — all the information is fed back to your own doctor.

Nurses

IVF nurses are registered nurses who're sometimes also qualified midwives or nurse practitioners. Before nurses can take on the responsibilities of IVF nursing they usually must have up to a year of training within an IVF clinic.

The nurses are the team members you see most often: They're the ones who hold your hand and guide you through the steps involved in IVF. IVF nurses are often called *nurse coordinators* because they make sure that all members of the team are lined up ready to go when you need them and that you know exactly what you need to do each day. During your treatment the nurses are your closest allies and you can always turn to them for information, instruction, advice, support and understanding.

In smaller clinics you often see the same nurse every time you're at the clinic, but in larger clinics you can expect to see a few different nursing faces during your treatment.

You may come across a nurse who you really get along with and who you feel is tuned in to you and your needs. If this happens, ask her whether she's willing to be 'your' nurse for the extent of your treatment (providing she's on duty when you need her, of course). Having one person who takes charge is easier for you because you don't have to repeat your story endlessly and you know who to turn to when you need support.

Counsellors

One of the conditions for getting a licence to open an IVF clinic is that couples who come for treatment have access to an IVF counsellor. IVF counsellors are counsellors, psychologists or social workers who specialise in the psychological aspects of infertility and infertility treatment and must be members of the Australian and New Zealand Infertility Counsellors Association (ANZICA).

The counsellor's job is to help you keep the stress of treatment at manageable levels and to be there to give you a boost of support if you need it. You can see the counsellor individually or as a couple, depending on what you feel is best for you. The counsellor can

- ✔ Explain things you don't understand
- ✔ Give you a heads-up on the common emotional reactions to IVF treatment and tips on how to deal with them
- ✔ Help you if you encounter relationship problems
- ✔ Talk you through any difficult decisions that you have to make

Counsellors are very useful people indeed and you should get in touch with one whenever you feel the need to. Speak to one of the nurses or reception staff if you want to see a counsellor and he or she will arrange an appointment for you.

Embryologists

Embryologists are highly specialised scientists who work in the IVF lab: Each IVF baby's life starts in their hands. Their skill, dedication and constant pursuit of improvements to IVF technology have dramatically improved the IVF success rate over the years.

The IVF lab has a scientific director who manages the embryologists and makes sure that all systems operate to perfection, so that the embryos that start life in the lab get the best possible chance to continue to develop.

The IVF lab is a sterile environment and staff who work there wear lab clothes and funny-looking paper hats. Don't let that put you off: If you have any lab-related questions, embryologists are usually more than happy to spend some time with you explaining what goes on in the lab. If you'd like to speak directly to an embryologist, talk to the reception staff or one of the nurses to arrange an appointment.

Pathologists

Pathologists examine all the blood specimens that you give during IVF treatment and report the results back to your IVF doctor. You're unlikely to meet the pathologists, but their importance in the IVF team needs to be acknowledged. The test results dictate how your treatment is managed, so your IVF doctor has to be completely confident that the results are correct.

Ultrasonographers

During your course of IVF you have several vaginal ultrasound examinations completed by an *ultrasonographer*. These specialists can decipher the strange-looking black-and-white images of your insides and provide your IVF doctor with a detailed report of how your treatment is progressing.

All being well, you'll meet the ultrasonographer again after treatment — for your first pregnancy scan!

Anaesthetists

Before your eggs are collected (see Chapter 5), an *anaesthetist* puts you to sleep so that you're 'out of it' and pain-free during the process, and hopefully feel fine when you wake up afterwards. In some clinics you can stay awake during egg collection, but an anaesthetist is present to give you something to help you relax.

Administration staff

Clinic administration staff help you through the jungle of paperwork and keep tabs of your appointments. The receptionist is usually a great source of information if you're looking for something or someone, and the people in the accounts department are experts at explaining the financial side of things.

Getting the most out of your team

Despite the number of people on your IVF team, ideally you should

- ✔ Be able to get hold of a team member easily when you need to
- ✔ Feel that all team members care about you and respond to your needs
- ✔ Feel well-informed and well-supported throughout your treatment
- ✔ Have confidence in the team members being knowledgeable and competent

In smaller clinics you soon get to know who's who and the team members get to know you quickly too, so communication usually flows easily. In larger clinics it can be more difficult to know who to turn to when you need information and support, but if the clinic is well run you're in good hands (even if there are many of them).

The following section includes some tips for getting the most out of your team.

When phoning the clinic, you may get frustrated sometimes trying to find the right person to talk to. You may find yourself being kept on hold (listening to music you don't even like) or being transferred from one person to another without getting anywhere. It may even be hard finding someone willing to talk to you. If this happens, put on your sternest voice and ask the receptionist to find someone to call you back within ten minutes (or whatever time frame you think is fair).

Looking for general information

Clinics usually have heaps of written information on most aspects of IVF that you can access either on the clinic website or as a hard copy from the clinic reception. If this material doesn't contain what you need, ask your IVF nurse to help or to point you in the right direction.

If your query is more specific — for example, you may want to know more about what causes male factor infertility, or look up IVF statistics for Australia or figure out how to find an egg donor — ask your IVF doctor.

Needing support

From time to time having IVF treatment gets tough and you may want to talk to someone or get advice about how to manage the stress (I explain more about coping with stress in IVF in Chapter 9). The most obvious first port of call is, of course, the counsellors, so feel free to call the clinic to make an appointment with a counsellor. If that's not soon enough for you and you need to offload straight away, your best bet is to contact one of the nurses, who're more than willing to listen to you and do their best to help.

You may find joining a support group helpful. The counsellors can put you in touch with the right people. Some larger clinics have support groups linked to them; the benefit is that group members share the experience of going through treatment at the same clinic.

Keeping up with your treatment progress

During treatment you keep in close contact with the IVF nurse either by phone or via email. The nurse informs you about your test results, tells you what to do next, schedules your appointments and hopefully gives you good news about the progress of your treatment.

If you need to know anything relating to your treatment, contact the nurse: If she doesn't have the answer to your question, she can find someone who does.

Seeking scientific information

The scientific side of IVF treatment is very complex, but you need to have some understanding of the process. At a minimum you need to grasp some facts about reproduction in general, how fertility drugs work (see Chapter 6) and early embryo development (see Chapter 7). Reading this book is a great start, but your IVF doctor and the embryologists are always willing to help you to get your head around the science of IVF.

Embryologists are the guardians of your precious eggs and sperm; they're the people you entrust to produce healthy embryos for you. When an embryologist has completed this task for you, he or she discusses the results with you and this often involves a fair bit of technical information about embryo development. Make sure that you understand the process; if you don't, ask the embryologist or your IVF doctor to carefully explain and keep asking questions until you know as much as possible about your embryos (sometimes a drawing makes it easier to understand).

Understanding costs and fees

Believe it or not, IVF billing can be one of the hardest things to understand because you need to keep tab of several transactions. You usually pay money upfront to the clinic when you start treatment and then some may be reimbursed to you by Medicare and/or your private health insurance fund. Most clinics have a member of staff dedicated to explaining the billing procedure and to help you follow the money trail.

Fixing a communication breakdown

Good communication between members of the IVF team (including you) is crucial to ensure a smooth journey through the IVF process, whether the treatment ultimately is successful or not. The IVF team can't always help a couple to have a baby, but team members can and should make sure that the couple are always treated in a compassionate, respectful and sensitive way.

However, the relationship between patients and doctors/other healthcare professionals can be pretty uneven, because patients are at the mercy of those who treat them and have to rely on the staff members' good intentions and professional expertise. Occasionally communication breaks down and you're caught in the middle. If that happens, don't suffer in silence.

When you experience problems with your IVF clinic you may not want to voice your complaints because you don't want to get a 'black dot' against your name or get a reputation for being 'difficult'. Think of IVF just like any other service you buy. If you stay at a hotel and the towels are dirty and the breakfast coffee is cold, wouldn't you complain to hotel management about the poor service? And wouldn't you complain to the mechanic if your car still wasn't working after you paid a lot of money to have it fixed? Similarly, if you're not happy with the care you receive when you have IVF, complain to the clinic.

Sometimes, you may have problems with one particular staff member. Try these options:

- If you feel that the 'chemistry' between you and one of the staff clashes and you just know that you're not on the same wavelength, don't put up with the situation. Make the point nicely but firmly to the person with whom you clash that you want someone else to look after you.

- When you experience difficulties in the way a staff member treats you or communicates with you, talking about the problem with a counsellor can help. Counsellors are expert at understanding how people relate to each other and you can trust them to help you deal with any difficulties you may have with clinic staff.

Putting pen to paper and making a formal written complaint is a sure way of drawing attention to a problem that may exist in a clinic. Try to be factual about what you see as the problem and offer some constructive advice about how you think it can be fixed. This can help the managers of the clinic to improve the standard of care and make life on IVF more bearable for you and your fellow patients.

Chapter 5

Taking IVF One Step at a Time

*1*VF treatment follows the stages of the menstrual cycle. That's why you hear people referring to a 'treatment cycle' or an 'IVF cycle' or sometimes just a 'cycle' when they describe the steps involved in an IVF attempt. You also hear clinic staff use weird acronyms for different types of treatment instead of the often very long and technical real names of these treatments.

An IVF cycle is like a series of hurdles that you have to jump over without falling. After you make it over one hurdle, another one is ahead of you. If you miss a hurdle, you go back to square one.

In this chapter, I explain all the strange acronyms involved in IVF. I also give you a detailed description of what you can expect in each step of a treatment cycle, why treatment sometimes doesn't go to plan and what your doctor may do to improve your chances if you have to try again.

Coming to Grips with All the IVF Acronyms and What They Mean

Several forms of treatment have evolved from the original IVF technique developed in the late 1970s. These treatments all go by their short names, or acronyms, with which you soon become familiar. Here's an explanation of what these acronyms mean and the treatments involved:

TECHNICAL STUFF

- ✔ **IVF, in-vitro fertilisation:** *In-vitro fertilisation* literally means 'fertilisation in glass' and the term was coined because in the early days the eggs and sperm were placed in glass test tubes where fertilisation and early embryo development took place (hence the name *test-tube baby*). These days, shallow plastic dishes are used instead, but the procedure remains much the same. The dish of eggs and sperm is placed in an incubator, which keeps the environment as close as possible to the conditions in a woman's body. All going well, after a few days the eggs fertilise and form embryos, and one or two of these embryos are placed in the woman's uterus.

- ✔ **ICSI, intracytoplasmic sperm injection:** IVF works only when the male partner has a normal or next-to-normal sperm count. (I tell you what's considered a normal sperm count in Chapter 1.) Scientists tried for a long time to work out how to help couples with male factor infertility and finally, in the early 1990s, they succeeded. ICSI helps many couples with male fertility problems. Instead of a sperm having to fight its way into the egg to fertilise it, the embryologist gives the sperm a helping hand. Using a so-called micro manipulator, the embryologist holds an egg still with a fine glass pipette called — you guessed it — a holding pipette. She or he then 'catches' a single sperm and injects it into the centre of the egg (the cytoplasm) using an extremely fine needle. The process from hereon is then the same as for IVF.

- ✔ **GIFT, gamete intrafallopian transfer:** GIFT was launched in the 1980s as a more 'natural' version of IVF. Instead of fertilisation happening outside the woman's body in a dish, the woman's eggs are retrieved from her ovaries and 'sandwiched' between two layers of sperm in fine tubing. This tubing is fed into one of the woman's fallopian tubes, where the eggs and sperm are left to fertilise.

  GIFT can be used only in couples with unexplained infertility but is rarely used these days, mainly because the woman undergoes a surgical procedure (laparoscopy) to place the eggs and sperm in her fallopian tube. However, GIFT can be an option for couples who don't want to use IVF for religious reasons, providing the woman's fallopian tubes are in working order.

- ✔ **PESA, percutaneous epididymal sperm aspiration, and MESA, microsurgical epididymal sperm aspiration:** Although some men produce sperm, the tubes that move the sperm from the testicles to the ejaculate may be either blocked or absent. Doctors can overcome this problem using one of two procedures to obtain sperm for ICSI:

  - • PESA: The doctor uses a needle to aspirate sperm-containing fluid from the epididymis, a duct on top of the testes where sperm is stored prior to ejaculation.

- MESA: The doctor extracts fluid from the epididymis by making a small incision in the scrotum.

The embryologist then locates the sperm in the fluid and performs ICSI.

✔ **PGD, pre-implantation genetic diagnosis:** Some families suffer genetic conditions that cause severe health problems. Embryologists can screen embryos to find the embryos that are free of the defective genes, allowing couples to use only the healthy embryos. (I discuss PGD in more detail in Chapter 16.)

✔ **TESA, testicular sperm aspiration, and TESE, testicular sperm extraction:** If a more severe male factor problem is evident, the doctor can perform one of two procedures to obtain sperm for ICSI:

- TESA: The doctor uses a fine needle to take microscopic pieces of tissue from the testis; this procedure is also called a testicular biopsy.

- TESE: The doctor surgically removes tissue from the testicles; this procedure is also called an open testicular biopsy.

The embryologist then dissects the small pieces of tissue under a microscope looking for sperm to use for ICSI.

Getting Started: Preliminary Tests and Paperwork

After completing the infertility investigation, you need to sort out a few preliminaries before you can start IVF treatment. These issues can take a few weeks to sort out, so make sure that you allow for this time on top of the four to six weeks you set aside for your first treatment cycle.

Completing some basic medical tests

You need to have several more medical tests before treatment can finally begin. These basic tests help your IVF doctor to manage your treatment effectively.

✔ **Screening blood tests:** Couples are routinely tested for several things, including:

- Blood group

- German measles (Rubella) and chickenpox (Varicella) immunity — only the female partner needs these tests; if you're not immune to these infectious diseases, you need to be immunised before starting treatment

- Hepatitis B and C
- HIV and syphilis

✔ **Other blood tests:** Depending on the cause of your infertility, you may need to have some of your hormone levels checked.

✔ **Sperm test:** Even if you've already had a sperm test, you may be asked to have another test done in a specialist lab where a more-detailed assessment of the quality of your sperm can be undertaken.

✔ **Ultrasound examinations:** Your eggs are collected via ultrasound, so an initial vaginal ultrasound examination allows your IVF doctor to see how accessible your ovaries are. Your doctor also uses the image to check the health of your ovaries and uterus, and determine the dose of fertility drugs that's best for you.

Undergoing counselling

Most clinics offer couples the opportunity to meet with an infertility counsellor before starting treatment — although in Victoria, this is actually required by law. Whether mandatory or not, many couples benefit from talking things over with a counsellor as part of preparing for treatment. Infertility counsellors are experts on the emotional aspects of infertility and infertility treatment and can offer you many useful tips on how to manage the stress of treatment.

Legally speaking

According to a guide to clinics published by the Victorian Infertility Treatment Authority, counsellors must discuss certain points with couples before they can have IVF treatment. For the purposes of section 11(1) of the *Infertility Treatment Act* (1995), counselling is required in relation to the following prescribed matters:

(a) *The options or choices available to the particular woman and her husband*

(b) *The law relating to infertility treatment in Victoria and the rights of the woman and her husband under that law*

(c) *The psychosocial and ethical issues related to infertility and infertility treatment*

(d) *The possible outcomes of an infertility treatment procedure, including the success rates of such treatment*

(e) *Any issue or concern raised by the woman or her husband in relation to the treatment procedure*

Consenting to treatment

As with other medical procedures, you have to give your permission for IVF treatment by signing consent forms. The exact content of the forms varies between clinics, but each form incorporates information about the procedures you agree to have and the risks of treatment, including the fact that the treatment may be unsuccessful.

You may also be asked to decide on the following:

- ✔ The number of embryos that can be transferred at any one time
- ✔ What you want to happen to any embryos that you don't need
- ✔ Whether you agree to have your embryos frozen
- ✔ Whether you agree to scientific research being performed on any embryos that aren't suitable for transfer or freezing

You and your partner need to agree on the choices you make, so take the forms home and discuss the options together, so that you're comfortable with what you sign.

Consent forms can be difficult to understand: Read the forms carefully and if anything seems unclear, ask your doctor to explain the details to you before you sign.

Finding out exactly what happens in an IVF cycle

At most clinics, the nurses make sure that you know what to do throughout the course of your IVF cycle. So, before you start your cycle, you have a scheduled appointment with a nurse to find out what to expect and what you need to do at each step. This meeting is likely to cover:

- ✔ The drugs used to stimulate egg production — and when and how you take them
- ✔ The potential side effects of these drugs
- ✔ How your response to the drugs is monitored
- ✔ Why these drugs sometimes don't work so well
- ✔ What happens on the day of egg retrieval
- ✔ When and how the sperm are collected

✔ What happens in the lab

✔ When you can expect to find out about the number of embryos you have

✔ What happens on the day the embryos are transferred

✔ What happens to any embryos that are frozen

✔ When to come back for a pregnancy test

✔ What happens after the pregnancy test

At the end of the meeting you receive this information in writing, so that you can refer back to the notes as and when you need to.

The nurse's job is to make sure that you have all the information you need before you start treatment. Sometimes, a nurse may be so keen to tell you everything at your first meeting that she forgets to ask what *you* want to know. The first appointment with the nurse is your best chance to get her full attention, so make sure you explain what's important to you so she understands your needs. Write down any questions you have before your appointment and ask the nurse to explain anything you don't understand.

Make a note of the name and contact details of the nurse you see for your initial appointment so that you can get in touch with her again directly when you need to.

Suffering information overload

The sheer volume of information that you have to take in before you undergo IVF treatment is huge. Naturally, you may worry about not remembering it all or getting something wrong. Make sure that you and your partner attend as many of the appointments as possible during your treatment, because between the two of you, you'll retain more information than either of you would on your own! And you can be sure that all the important stuff you need to know is included in the written information that the nurse gives you to take home, so, if in doubt, refer to your paperwork.

Producing Mature Eggs with Fertility Drugs

Historically, IVF treatment used a woman's one and only egg that normally develops during the monthly menstrual cycle. The chances of getting this egg before ovulation and of fertilisation occurring normally were very slim, which is why the chance of pregnancy was very low. These days, the clinic uses fertility drugs to stimulate your ovaries to produce multiple eggs as well as other drugs to stop the eggs from ovulating, which increases the chance of at least one of your eggs developing into an embryo that has all it takes to grow into a healthy baby.

Women's responses to fertility drugs vary: Some women produce a lot of eggs while others produce only a few. Your age and genetic factors influence the number of eggs that you can expect, but your doctor can't possibly predict in advance the number of eggs that will be collected. However, your doctor can estimate your *ovarian reserve* before starting stimulation by measuring your levels of follicle-stimulating hormone (FSH) and anti-müllerian hormone (AMH) and examining your ovaries with ultrasound. The ovarian reserve gives your doctor some idea of what to expect and can help determine the most suitable dose of fertility drugs to use.

But even when your doctor carefully considers your individual circumstances to determine your dose of fertility drugs, ovarian stimulation doesn't always go to plan and you sometimes end up with too few or too many eggs.

I discuss the drugs used in IVF in more detail in Chapter 6.

Stimulating your ovaries

To understand the IVF process, ideally you need to be familiar with the relevant parts of the menstrual cycle, so here's a quick recap on how eggs are normally formed in your body. The pituitary gland in your brain regulates your menstrual cycle by producing two hormones: *follicle-stimulating hormone (FSH)* and *luteinising hormone (LH)*. Your pituitary gland releases follicle-stimulating hormone which, as the name suggests, stimulates the growth of several *follicles* in your ovaries. Follicles are fluid-filled sacks and each follicle contains one egg. As the follicles grow, one becomes dominant and the other follicles stop developing. When the dominant follicle reaches a certain size, your pituitary gland releases luteinising hormone, which causes the egg to mature and leads to *ovulation*, when the follicle bursts and releases the egg. Your fallopian tube captures the egg, which may then be fertilised.

The drugs that are used in IVF 'trick' your body into bringing to maturity *multiple* follicles and eggs and then stop the eggs from ovulating too soon so that in-vitro fertilisation can take place.

You receive daily injections of follicle-stimulating hormone to promote the growth of multiple follicles. When the follicles reach a certain size you have a single injection of *human chorionic gonadotrophin (hCG)* to trigger the final maturation of the eggs.

To prevent the follicles from releasing the eggs too soon, most controlled ovarian stimulation protocols include a class of drugs called *gonadotrophin-releasing hormone (GnRH) analogues*, given as either a nasal spray or an injection. This drug blocks the body's normal production of follicle-stimulating hormone and luteinising hormone from the pituitary gland, and makes sure the eggs aren't released before the egg collection procedure.

You receive your injections of follicle-stimulating hormone *subcutaneously*, meaning just under the skin, with a short needle. Since you need these injections on a daily basis, the most convenient method is for you to give yourself the injections, and the nurse shows you exactly how to do this.

If you find it too difficult to inject yourself, the nurse can show your partner or a friend how to give you the injections.

After a week or so of injecting yourself with follicle-stimulating hormone, you probably feel a bit like a pincushion, but your injection technique should be down pat. Now's the time to attend your scheduled vaginal ultrasound examination to find out how your ovaries are responding to the drugs. From the ultrasound image, your doctor can:

- Check your ovaries close up to count and measure the size of the follicles that are growing.
- Measure the thickness of the lining in your uterus, which is an important indicator of how 'ready' the eggs are.

Looking at the ultrasound image, you may see a few bigger follicles and many small follicles. Bear in mind that the number of follicles you see on ultrasound is *not* necessarily the same as the number of eggs you end up with, because:

- Only the big follicles contain mature eggs.
- The eggs can be hard to find, so counting the number of bigger follicles doesn't necessarily equal the number of eggs you get.

In addition to the ultrasound, you may be asked to have a blood test to measure the level of *oestradiol* (a hormone produced by growing follicles) in your body.

Putting together the information from the ultrasound examination and the blood test helps your doctor to decide how many more days of follicle-stimulating hormone injections you need and whether the dose should be increased or decreased.

Breaking the menopause myth

Will I reach menopause sooner because I 'use up' so many eggs in IVF?

Many women who use fertility drugs and produce a lot of eggs ask this question. Women become menopausal when they run out of eggs, and since in a normal menstrual cycle only one egg ovulates, the question is a fair one for women on IVF producing many eggs. Fortunately, IVF stimulation does *not* shorten your ovaries' active life. Here's why:

✔ In a normal cycle, several follicles begin to grow but over time one takes the lead to become the dominant follicle and produce

a mature egg at ovulation. All the other follicles are spent and lose their chance to ever produce an egg.

✔ In a stimulated cycle, the fertility drugs rescue the follicles that would've been spent in a normal cycle and allow many of them to grow and reach the stage where they contain a mature egg.

So you produce the *same number* of eggs in a stimulated cycle as in a normal cycle: The difference is that in a stimulated cycle more of them reach maturity.

Maturing the eggs

You may undergo additional ultrasound examinations or blood tests over the next few days to determine when the eggs are ready to be fertilised. When the largest follicles reach a diameter of 18 mm or more, the lining in your uterus is thickening well and your oestradiol levels are still rising, the time to collect your eggs is getting close.

Before eggs and sperm can finally meet, the eggs have to be matured and for this you have an injection of *human chorionic gonadotrophin (hCG)*, which acts like luteinising hormone to prompt maturation of the eggs. The injection is scheduled between 34 and 37 hours before the planned egg collection. The timing of the injection usually works out to be late in the evening two days before your eggs are due to be collected.

The nurse tells you the exact time for your injection and is sure to carry on a bit about the importance of sticking to this schedule — for a good reason:

✔ Receive your dose of hCG too late and your eggs won't get enough exposure to it, so they may not be perfectly mature when they're collected.

✔ Receive your dose of hCG too early and, even worse, the eggs may not be available when the doctor tries to collect them, because hCG also triggers ovulation after the eggs are mature.

Understanding what can go wrong with stimulation

No-one can predict exactly how you (or any woman) may respond to the fertility drugs you're given on your first IVF cycle. For most women the response is sufficient to proceed to the next hurdle — egg collection. But in 10 to 15 per cent of cases, treatment in the first cycle may end with stimulation because either not enough or too many follicles are seen on ultrasound, or the oestradiol level isn't quite right (see the section 'Stimulating your ovaries' earlier in the chapter).

- If very few follicles are evident, the chance of getting eggs is low, so your doctor may suggest cancelling the cycle and trying again with a higher dose of drugs.

- If more than 20 follicles are seen, you may be at risk of *ovarian hyperstimulation syndrome* (OHSS). (I explain the nasty nature of this extreme response to the drugs in Chapter 10.) If your doctor thinks that continuing the cycle is too risky, he or she may advise you not to go ahead with egg collection and start a new cycle with a lower dose of drugs.

In addition, sometimes problems are unearthed when you have the ultrasound examination. For example:

- The signs may indicate that the best time for egg collection has passed.

- You may have a cyst on your ovary, which can mess up your hormone levels. Your doctor will talk to you about what that means in terms of future treatment, but these cysts are generally harmless and disappear with time. You may be asked to have an ultrasound and/or hormone tests before trying again.

Collecting the Eggs

If you respond well to the stimulating part of the IVF cycle, you're over the first hurdle! The next step is egg collection, which is a relatively simple and quick procedure.

The nurse tells you what time you need to arrive for admission, when your surgery is scheduled and when you can expect to be discharged. You must fast before surgery — that is, have nothing to eat or drink — starting the night before admission. And you must show up without make-up and nail polish — very unglamorous.

Even though egg collection doesn't take long, don't plan to do anything else on the day you have the surgery because you may not be up for it.

You can't drive in the 24 hours after the egg collection because the anaesthetic can affect your coordination, so arrange for someone to take you home.

Undergoing the egg collection procedure

After weeks of injections, the big day for you and your partner finally arrives. You're bound to feel nervous. In fact, probably all sorts of emotions are churning around inside you.

You receive a light general anaesthetic for your egg collection procedure, and the trusted ultrasound machine is used for collection. The ultrasound probe is covered with a sterile plastic cover and fitted with a needle guide, along which a long metal needle slides. The surgery proceeds as follows (see also Figure 5-1):

1. The doctor inserts the ultrasound probe into your vagina to locate the follicles in your ovaries.

2. When your doctor has a clear view of a follicle he or she punctures it with the needle through the vaginal wall and sucks the follicular fluid into a test tube.

3. The doctor continues this process until all visible follicles are punctured and the follicular fluid is collected in test tubes.

4. The test tubes are passed to the lab where the embryologist tips the fluid into a dish and looks for the eggs under a microscope. The lab is usually adjacent to the theatre and the embryologist keeps your doctor up to speed with the egg tally.

The procedure usually takes only 15 to 20 minutes and then you're wheeled into a recovery area where you wake up soon afterwards. When you're 'with it' the doctor tells you how many eggs were found.

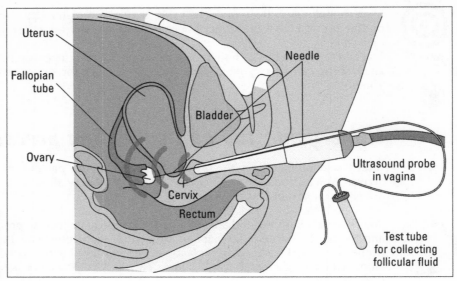

Figure labels: Uterus, Fallopian tube, Ovary, Cervix, Rectum, Bladder, Needle, Ultrasound probe in vagina, Test tube for collecting follicular fluid

Recovering from the egg collection procedure

An hour or two after your egg collection, you get a bite to eat and then you're ready to go home. Before you leave, you're given details about when to contact the IVF clinic to find out if and how many of your eggs have fertilised and when you're needed back for embryo transfer. In most clinics you call the nurses for this information.

Take it easy for a day or two after your egg collection. You're bound to experience cramping and feel a bit sore afterwards, and some vaginal bleeding from the needle perforations is to be expected.

You can use painkillers if you need to after the egg collection procedure but make sure that you use paracetamol, not aspirin, because aspirin has a blood-thinning effect, which can increase the bleeding from the puncture sites. When in doubt, ask your IVF doctor about which medications to use.

Getting fewer eggs than expected

Ideally, you have eight to twelve eggs and you and your partner are mightily relieved, because the more eggs that are collected, the greater your chance of having a baby. But what happens when you have only a couple of eggs — or worse, none at all?

Obviously, if you expect to get ten eggs and get only two, you may be disappointed. But this doesn't mean the end of the cycle — you can still progress to the next stage.

Finding no eggs is a devastating outcome that very rarely happens, but when it does this obviously means the end of the treatment cycle. If this happens you need to have a serious discussion with your doctor to find out whether this was just bad luck or is likely to happen again. This discussion can help you decide whether to try again with another treatment cycle.

Ultrasound guided egg retrieval is a simple and safe procedure. I discuss the rare possible risks involved in having the egg collection procedure in Chapter 10.

Obtaining the Sperm

In most cases getting the sperm doesn't involve sharp needles, but sometimes it does. The method used for obtaining the sperm depends on whether sperm are present in the ejaculate or not.

Producing a sperm sample

If you have viable sperm in the ejaculate, you're asked to produce a sperm sample on the day of your partner's egg collection. You're shown to a private room designed for the purpose where you produce the sample.

The infertility investigation inevitably involves a sperm test, so you should have had a chance to practise ejaculating into a small plastic jar before the big day! However, when the pressure is on, ejaculating can be difficult. If you have an inkling that this may happen to you, speak to your doctor or nurse before the sperm sample is needed and they can discuss alternatives to make sure that sperm is available on the day of egg collection:

✔ Produce the sample at home and bring it to the clinic if you live within an hour or so from the clinic, or you can use a hotel room close to the clinic.

✔ Freeze a sample ahead of time and use it for back-up, just in case. Sometimes, knowing that you have a back-up sample in the freezer is enough to relieve anxiety, so freezing sperm to lift the pressure can be a good idea. (See the section 'Freezing sperm in advance' later in the chapter.)

✔ Ask your partner to help you, but do this before egg collection because your partner could be too sleepy or sore after her egg collection.

✔ Ask your doctor to prescribe Viagra for you, which can help you to overcome performance anxiety.

Don't use lubricants when you masturbate, because they kill the sperm.

Embryologists recommend two to four days of abstinence before you produce sperm for IVF treatment because:

✔ Avoiding ejaculation for a long time before the sample is needed can make the sperm quality *worse*: So no, you can't improve the quality of your sperm by 'saving up' for a long time before the sample is needed.

✔ Ejaculating too close to the time when the sperm sample is needed may *reduce* the number of sperm in the ejaculate.

Freezing sperm in advance

As long as your sperm tests are normal you can produce a sample in advance to be kept frozen until the day of egg collection. You may prefer this option if you worry about having difficultly producing a sample on the day it's needed or if you work away from home for long periods of time: Rather than trying to coordinate work and treatment schedules, stored sperm can be thawed on the day of egg collection.

Retrieving sperm surgically

If you have no sperm in the ejaculate (refer to Chapter 1), the sperm are retrieved via a surgical procedure under local or general anaesthesia. Depending on what type of infertility you have, the doctor retrieves either fluid or microscopic pieces of tissue from the testicles. I explain these procedures in the section 'Coming to Grips with All the IVF Acronyms and What They Mean' earlier in this chapter. Depending on the clinic and the type of procedure you're having, you may be asked not to eat or drink anything starting the night before your surgery.

If you have a general anaesthetic for the procedure, you can't drive for 24 hours afterwards, so you need to arrange for someone to take you home. You may feel a bit bruised and sore after the anaesthetic wears off, but this pain eases over a couple of days.

Finding solutions to a poor sperm sample

Occasionally, the quality of the sperm produced on the day of egg collection is unexpectedly poor. This can happen if you had an episode of high fever some weeks beforehand but can also be part of the normal variations in sperm quality. If this happens to you and you were planning to have IVF, your doctor may suggest trying intracytoplasmic sperm injection as an alternative procedure (I explain this procedure in the section 'Coming to Grips with All the IVF Acronyms and What They Mean' earlier in this chapter). If you go ahead with this alternative procedure, there's a good chance the eggs may fertilise.

Very rarely, either you may not be able to produce sperm or no sperm are found in your ejaculate. Unfortunately, the eggs can't wait very long for sperm, so if no sperm are available on the day the eggs are collected, the eggs won't fertilise without a rescue operation. If this happens to you, these are the rescue options:

- ✔ If you have frozen sperm stored as back-up, this can be used.

- ✔ Your doctor may try to extract sperm directly from your testicles using a needle. If this procedure works, the embryologist can perform intracytoplasmic sperm injection.

- ✔ The embryologist may offer to freeze the eggs and keep them stored until some sperm can be extracted. However, eggs don't freeze very well, so this option offers only a very small chance of rescuing the cycle.

Giving Nature a Hand

After the eggs and sperm are safely delivered to the capable embryologists in the lab, you have to rely on their expertise and a good dose of luck for the next few days. In Chapter 7, I explain in detail what happens in the lab, but all being well, over the next few days eggs and sperm magically transform into healthy embryos.

All the equipment that's used in the lab where your eggs, sperm and embryos are kept is carefully labelled with your details to make sure that no mix-ups occur. I discuss the systems in place to avoid mix-ups in Chapter 7.

Performing magic in the lab

After selecting the mature eggs and cleaning the sperm, the embryologists start their part in the magic by adding a droplet with thousands of sperm to each egg if you're having IVF, or by injecting a single sperm into each egg if you're having intracytoplasmic sperm injection. Each egg/sperm combination is kept in a dish in a special culture medium that has all the nutrients and trace elements embryos need to develop. The dishes are placed in an incubator where the environment mimics the inside of your fallopian tubes (where fertilisation normally happens). In most cases the magic works and fertilisation takes place so that after a few days the first stages of embryo development have taken place.

In the meantime, of course, you're biting your fingernails at home waiting to find out whether you're over the next hurdle! The embryologists can see whether any eggs are fertilised the day after egg collection, so call the clinic the day after your surgery to find out how many of your eggs are fertilised. The clinic staff also tell you what time your embryo transfer is scheduled for.

Bear in mind that not all eggs fertilise normally and that the eggs that fertilise don't always continue to develop to healthy-looking embryos. So even if you start with a large number of eggs, some may not fertilise and of those that do, some may not continue to the cleavage stage.

Facing up to what can go wrong

For some women, the treatment cycle results in no fertilised eggs and bitter disappointment. Such a devastating result is hard to digest and you're anxious to find out why it happened. In most cases, the reason for abnormal fertilisation or embryo arrest can't be pinpointed, but it's most likely due to defects in the egg or sperm — or both.

Occasionally, none of the eggs fertilise normally or none of the fertilised eggs develop into a healthy embryo and the IVF cycle comes to an end. Each egg has a two in three chance of fertilising normally, so the fewer eggs you have, the greater the risk of zero fertilisation. This is what can happen:

- ✔ If you have IVF, occasionally more than one sperm gets into an egg and even if this egg then keeps developing, it can't be used because it's chromosomally abnormal.

- ✔ Whether you have IVF or ICSI, eggs sometimes don't fertilise.

- ✔ Occasionally, normally fertilised eggs don't continue their development or embryos that have formed stop developing. Embryos that stop developing aren't viable and can't be used.

Transferring the Embryos

Assuming all goes well, the next hurdle is embryo transfer. When you arrive at the clinic for transfer your doctor gives you the latest update on the development of your embryos and advises whether any embryos are available for freezing. Your doctor explains

- How many embryos have developed normally
- The quality of your embryos as assessed by the embryologist (see Chapter 7)
- How many embryos can be frozen (see Chapter 7)

If possible, both you and your partner should attend the clinic because you may well need each other to help take in all this information. Plus, embryo transfer is such a special moment in an IVF cycle, you'll want to share the experience.

Even if you have more than one embryo available for transfer, most clinics recommend that only one embryo be transferred. Your doctor will explain the pros and cons of having two embryos transferred depending on your age and the quality of your embryos. Basically, however, transferring two embryos:

- May slightly increase your chance of pregnancy
- Definitely increases your risk of having twins

So, you need to weigh up the risk of having twins (which I explain in Chapter 10) against the possibility of a small increase in your chance of becoming pregnant if two embryos are transferred.

However, your doctor may recommend transferring two embryos in the following circumstances:

- The embryologists judge that the embryos have a slightly reduced chance of survival.
- You're over 38 years of age and/or have already had several unsuccessful IVF attempts.

Reducing the risk of multiple births

In the early days of IVF each patient had all her available embryos transferred at the same time, since each embryo had a very slim chance of surviving and the technique of freezing embryos hadn't been worked out. Yet the chance of pregnancy was still extremely low. However, over time laboratory techniques improved and embryos had a greater chance of surviving. In the 1980s and early 1990s, IVF often hit the headlines when record multiple births were reported. Between 1982 and 1990 the number of triplets and quadruplets born in Australia tripled.

This trend caused concern among obstetricians and paediatricians because of the greater risks of multiple births to mothers and babies. In 1988 the Fertility Society of Australia, the professional society for practitioners in IVF, recommended that no more than three embryos be transferred in any one cycle.

Today, the Reproductive Technology Accreditation Committee, the body that sets the standards for Australian IVF clinics, identifies as one of its priorities a reduction in the number of multiple births, including twins, resulting from IVF. The committee recommends that only one embryo be transferred in women under 35 and no more than two in women aged between 35 and 40.

Making the transfer

Embryo transfer is a rather simple procedure that takes only a few minutes and is about as painful as a PAP smear. Some clinics have a TV screen mounted in the transfer room so that you and your partner can glimpse the embryo as it's about to be transferred. Seeing the very first stages of human development is pretty exciting — you'll find the image stays with you.

The transfer proceeds as follows:

1. Your doctor places a speculum (a metal or plastic instrument to aid viewing) in your vagina and gently cleans your cervix.

2. The embryologist draws the embryo into a thin catheter (a hollow plastic tube) and your doctor passes the catheter through your cervix into your uterus. You may experience some discomfort when the catheter passes through your cervix, but it soon passes.

3. When the catheter is in place, your doctor carefully injects the embryo into your uterus and then removes the catheter.

The embryologist takes the catheter back to the lab and checks it under a microscope to make sure that the embryo was deposited in your uterus and is no longer in the catheter.

You don't need to rest after the transfer but before you go home the nurse gives you instructions about the hormone medication that you need to take to make sure that your progesterone levels remain high over the next couple of weeks. Your progesterone levels need to remain high to stop a period from starting before your embryo has had a chance to implant. Clinic protocols vary regarding the medication you take: You may be given human chorionic gonadotrophin injections or vaginal progesterone gel or pessaries. (For more detailed information about these drugs, see Chapter 6.)

Looking after yourself post-embryo transfer

You can now go home and live life as usual. Right! As if you'll be able to focus on anything but your embryo and what may be for the next few weeks.

Although you may be tempted to think that if you rest or reduce your physical activity to a minimum, you can improve the chance of the embryo 'taking', no evidence exists to show that resting makes any difference. And, if you feel up to it, having sex is fine too. So, you need take no particular precautions.

If you think of yourself as *potentially pregnant*, it makes sense to follow a healthy lifestyle and look after yourself. It may also be a good idea to avoid very strenuous activities — if only to avoid blaming yourself if the embryo transfer isn't ultimately successful.

Enduring the Longest Wait

Whether you've transferred fresh or frozen embryos, the next step is to go home, carry on with your normal activities and have a pregnancy test about two weeks later. As if that's possible!

What you really need to do is to brace yourself for the longest wait of your life, because during the two weeks there won't be a waking moment when your mind isn't busy thinking about your uterus. Every study about the IVF experience that I'm aware of has found that the hardest part is the wait after embryo transfer to find out whether the treatment has worked. It beats hands down the pain of injections, the intrusiveness of vaginal ultrasound examinations and the disruption of frequent clinic visits.

Up until embryo transfer, you're busy with injections, blood tests, ultrasounds, phone calls to the clinic, talking to the nurses and getting over all those early hurdles. Then, after embryo transfer, that last hurdle takes *so long* to get over — and all you can do is wait, wait, wait, and hope that you get over it. It's a nerve-wracking time because, whichever way it goes, the outcome undoubtedly has a profound impact on your life.

Looking for signs

You've no doubt heard how pregnant women have all sorts of signs and symptoms as soon as they conceive and how they just *know* that they're pregnant. These signs may be anything from tender breasts, nausea, tiredness and dizziness to needing to go to the toilet ten times every night. So, after transfer, you're looking for all these and other 'sure' signs of pregnancy. But, trust me, you can have all sorts of sure signs and not be pregnant, and you can be pregnant with no signs at all.

You may be very tempted to take a home pregnancy test to avoid the long wait. Unfortunately, home pregnancy tests require a fair amount of pregnancy hormone to be present in your urine to turn positive and enough won't develop in the first two weeks after embryo transfer. As a result, home test results during this time are often negative, even if you're pregnant.

Vaginal bleeding can be bad news if you're pregnant, so after IVF you can be forgiven for obsessively checking your underwear. But remember, spotting or light bleeding can happen when the embryo implants in the uterus, so such a sign isn't necessarily the end of the world. And even if you have slightly heavier bleeding, you may still be pregnant, so continue with any medication until you have the result of your pregnancy test. When in doubt, talk to your IVF doctor or nurse.

If you haven't had any bleeding at all by the time you have your pregnancy test, you may be pregnant. But a word of caution: Some of the hormone medications that you may take after embryo transfer can delay the onset of a period, so you need to wait for the result of your test to know whether the treatment has worked.

Staying sane

With so much at stake, you inevitably feel preoccupied and at the point of going crazy during this agonising two-week wait. Feeling tense and stressed during this time is normal and you have to manage as best you can. How you do this depends on who you are and what works for you. Some women prefer to keep busy with work or other demands, while others function better if they're free of outside pressures.

Some (perhaps even most) women feel better if they can talk to someone about the things that weigh on their mind, whereas men often feel better if they *don't* talk about them. If you find that you and your partner have different ways of getting through the angst of the two-week wait, try to find ways to handle the situation that work for each of you. For instance, your sister, mum, friend or the clinic counsellor may be able to act as a source of support for you if you and your partner have difficulty tackling this trying time together.

Understanding what can go wrong after embryo transfer

This last hurdle is the most difficult one to get over because, of all the embryos that are transferred, only some have what it takes to grow and develop into a healthy baby. Of course, this is true not only for IVF treatment but also for many spontaneously conceived pregnancies. Many pregnancies are lost at a very early stage, often even before the woman knows that she's pregnant. It's not uncommon for women to have a 'late' period delayed by a pregnancy that didn't continue beyond the first couple of weeks after conception.

However, while couples who can conceive spontaneously can try again to become pregnant without too much effort, couples who need IVF have to start the whole process again or have another transfer of frozen embryos if they have any stored.

Arriving at D-day: Your Pregnancy Test

Hard as it may be to believe, the day for your long-awaited pregnancy test does eventually arrive. For this test, most clinics require you to have a blood test, either at the clinic or locally if you live far from the clinic. The blood test measures the level of pregnancy hormone, β-hCG (beta human chorionic gonadotrophin), in your blood. Thankfully, the result is usually available later the same day and your IVF nurse gives you the news.

A positive pregnancy test marks the happy ending of a treatment cycle and the beginning of a pregnancy; a negative pregnancy test confirms that the IVF cycle was unsuccessful. Occasionally, the pregnancy test is indefinite, which means that the gruelling wait for answers continues.

A positive pregnancy test

If your test is positive, you, your partner and the nurse who gives you the result will be jumping for joy — you've cleared the final hurdle of the IVF obstacle course!

Some women already have an inkling that they're pregnant, but others find it hard to believe because they don't feel different in any way. And you may find that just as you breathe a sigh of relief that the worry of your treatment outcome is finally behind you, a new worry creeps in: Will the baby be okay? Such worries are quite normal and I explain how to handle them in Chapter 18.

The nurse arranges for you to have your first ultrasound examination about two weeks after your pregnancy test. If the early pregnancy is going well and a foetal heartbeat is seen at this examination, the IVF clinic refers you on to an antenatal clinic or a private obstetrician for pregnancy care (see Chapter 18).

Unfortunately, a few women get bad news when they have their ultrasound examination: I explain the risks of miscarriage and other types of pregnancy loss after IVF in Chapter 10.

A negative pregnancy test

A negative pregnancy test result is a terrible let-down. Your hopes are dashed after all the effort, time and money you've put in and you're back where you started. In Chapter 12 I talk about how to move on and make decisions about the future when treatment doesn't work.

An equivocal pregnancy test

Occasionally, the pregnancy test is indefinite, which means that the level of pregnancy hormone is lower than expected. This can be due to a number of factors:

- ✔ The embryo implanted and started to produce pregnancy hormone but didn't have all that it takes to continue to grow and develop.

- ✔ The embryo had a chromosomal abnormality that isn't compatible with life.

- ✔ The embryo implanted in the wrong place. This is called an *ectopic pregnancy* and I explain this potentially life-threatening situation in more detail in Chapter 10.

- ✔ The part of the embryo that makes the placenta is growing and producing pregnancy hormone but there is no foetus. This is called a *blighted ovum* and I explain this phenomenon in Chapter 10.

- ✔ Pregnancy hormone may be present in your blood for a couple of weeks even if the pregnancy doesn't continue to grow.

- ✔ Sometimes the pregnancy may be a bit 'slow' at getting going and embryologists talk about 'delayed implantation', which can explain lower-than-expected pregnancy hormone levels.

The fact that there is a measurable level of pregnancy hormone means that the embryo kept developing after it was transferred. However, you need to undergo more blood tests and perhaps an ultrasound examination before your doctor can tell you whether the pregnancy is continuing or not. This means that the endless wait for answers drags on and understandably you may find this limbo situation very difficult.

Having the Bonus of Frozen Embryos

The techniques for freezing *eggs* haven't yet been perfected (see Chapter 15) but scientists have developed very successful methods for freezing and thawing *embryos* (see Chapter 7). After a stimulated cycle, extra embryos are sometimes available that the embryologist judges as good quality and these embryos can be frozen for later transfers. Depending on how many embryos you have, these extra frozen embryos give you bonus chances of getting pregnant without having to go through all the hormone injections again!

Embryos can be kept frozen for many years, so if you fall pregnant after a stimulated cycle you can use your frozen embryos to have a second (or third or fourth . . .) baby if you want. If you don't fall pregnant after the stimulated cycle, you can use your frozen embryos as soon as you're ready. Some lucky couples complete their family with a single 'batch' of embryos: One clinic website mentions a couple who've had four children, one at a time, from the one stimulated cycle.

One of the critical parts of a frozen embryo transfer cycle is getting the transfer timing right. To maximise the chance of an embryo implanting, it needs to be transferred when the lining in the uterus is just right for implantation.

✔ If you have a *regular* menstrual cycle, the clinic monitors your cycle to determine when you ovulate, because just after ovulation is the right time to transfer the embryo. So, to use a frozen embryo, you contact the clinic on the first day of your period and the nurses tell you when to start monitoring ovulation, which in most clinics involves the following:

• A few days before ovulation is expected you have an ultrasound examination to check the size of the largest follicle and measure the thickness of the lining in the uterus, which are clues to when you're likely to ovulate.

• When you're close to ovulation you also have either daily blood or urine tests to detect the surge of luteinising hormone, which happens about a day before ovulation.

• Embryo transfer is scheduled three to five days after this luteinising hormone surge, depending on the stage at which the embryos were frozen.

✔ If you have an *irregular* menstrual cycle and it's difficult to know if or when you ovulate, you need to either complete an *artificial cycle* or have some hormone stimulation to make you ovulate. Both these methods aim to make the lining in your uterus suitable for implantation.

To complete an artificial cycle, you take medication to mimic the hormones produced by the ovaries in a normal menstrual cycle:

• You start by taking oestrogen tablets, which help grow the uterine lining.

• Ten to 14 days later you have an ultrasound examination to measure the thickness of the lining in your uterus.

• When the lining reaches a certain thickness (in most clinics this means 8 mm or more), you take progesterone in the form of injections, vaginal gel or pessaries.

• Embryo transfer is scheduled a few days after you start the progesterone.

• You must keep taking oestrogen and progesterone until the day of your pregnancy test and continue until week ten of the pregnancy if you're pregnant.

To help you to ovulate in preparation for transfer of frozen embryos your doctor:

• Prescribes a course of clomid tablets or FSH injections (see Chapter 6)

• Monitors follicle growth via ultrasound

- Asks you to have daily blood or urine tests when you're close to ovulating until the tests show a surge of luteinising hormone, which happens about one day before ovulation

- Schedules embryo transfer three to five days after this surge of luteinising hormone, depending on the stage at which your embryos were frozen

In a natural cycle, you may get a period before you have your pregnancy test if the treatment hasn't worked. This is because the progesterone level drops if the embryo doesn't implant — which triggers the period to start. But in an artificial cycle you continue to take progesterone until the day of your pregnancy test, so the level doesn't drop and the period isn't triggered if the embryo hasn't implanted. As a result, if you've completed an artificial cycle you need to keep your cool and wait for the results of your pregnancy test before getting too hopeful. Even if your period doesn't start before the pregnancy test, the treatment may not have worked.

Report *immediately* to the nurses any bleeding you have, because bleeding may indicate that your progesterone levels are too low and need to be topped up with additional progesterone pessaries, gel or injections.

Chapter 6

Taking Drugs, Drugs and More Drugs

Drugs are an inevitable part of IVF treatment. The goal of treatment is to make your ovaries produce several eggs all at once rather than the one egg you normally release every month. When you undergo treatment you're likely to feel like a pincushion and have hormones coming out of your ears, but using drugs give you a much better chance of success than attempting to get pregnant drug-free, because with treatment *every* egg has a small chance of being *the* egg. And the more eggs you produce, the greater your chance of falling pregnant.

In this chapter, I explain the various drugs used in IVF and what kinds of side effects you may experience — conveniently, any mood swings you get during IVF can be blamed on the drugs. I also discuss the factors that can influence how your ovaries respond to the drugs and how stimulation protocols can be individualised to your needs.

Understanding What Drugs Are Used, and Why

The main aim of IVF treatment is to make the most of every 'go'. So, while you normally release only one egg every month, which may or may not be 'perfect', with IVF the goal is to have about a dozen eggs reach maturity to improve the chance of at least one of them being 'just right'. To stimulate your ovaries to produce multiple eggs, your doctor gives you a carefully measured cocktail of drugs that can make you feel quite hormonal and a bit off the planet — but not in the same way as you feel after a few gin and tonics!

In this section I describe what you may find in your cocktail. Refer to Chapter 5 for more about hormone stimulation.

The contraceptive pill (strange, but true)

Who'd have thought that you need to take the *contraceptive pill* when you're trying to have a baby? Of course, there's a good reason for this. When you take the pill, your own hormones are put on hold and you don't ovulate (that's the whole point of taking the pill). So, a month or so before you start IVF treatment your doctor may prescribe the pill to suppress your own hormones in preparation for the drugs you need to take later to stimulate your ovaries.

Suppressing your own hormones in this way has two benefits:

- ✔ The hormone stimulation may be more effective.
- ✔ Scheduling treatment is easier. Because you're hormonally on hold when you take the pill, you and your doctor can choose a time to start the hormone stimulation that suits you both, rather than waiting for your period to start.

Your doctor gives you a prescription for the pill, which you can fill at any pharmacy. Your IVF nurse gives you instructions on how and when to take the pill.

Follicle-stimulating hormone

Follicle-stimulating hormone (FSH) promotes follicle growth. Follicles are the fluid-filled cysts in the ovaries where the eggs develop and mature. You take the drug in the form of a daily injection for as few as six days to possibly up to two weeks (and rarely more) if the dose has to be increased. The dose required to grow between 10 and 15 follicles varies between women: Your doctor calculates your dose and then may increase or decrease this amount depending on how your body responds.

The most common side effects of FSH are

- ✔ Abdominal discomfort
- ✔ Feeling bloated
- ✔ Influenza-like symptoms (rare)
- ✔ Irritability

Believe it or not

After menopause women still produce FSH, but since they have no follicles or eggs in their ovaries the hormone is simply excreted in their urine. Originally, drug companies used to produce FSH for fertility treatment by extracting the hormone from postmenopausal women's urine. The hormone was purified and turned into powdered form. The quality of this drug varied between batches and there was an element of uncertainty about its purity and exact bioactivity. These days synthetic FSH is produced using DNA technology, which means that the end product is uncontaminated and batches don't differ in bioactivity.

Another improvement is that today the drug is given subcutaneously with a tiny needle just under the skin, whereas the original product had to be given deep into the muscle with a huge needle.

✔ Irritation at the injection site

✔ Over-response, which can lead to ovarian hyperstimulation syndrome (OHSS) (I explain OHSS in Chapter 10)

✔ Tender breasts

FSH for IVF is provided for free under Medicare's Pharmaceutical Benefits Scheme (PBS) — which is great, because this drug is very expensive. Refer to Chapter 3 for more about the PBS.

Gonadotrophin-releasing hormone analogues

Gonadotrophin-releasing hormone (GnRH) is produced naturally in an area of the brain called the hypothalamus. This hormone controls the production of the two hormones that regulate the menstrual cycle: follicle-stimulating hormone and luteinising hormone (I explain how these hormones operate in Chapter 5). When you have IVF, the last thing you want to do is ovulate all the eggs that you've worked so hard to produce before your doctor has a chance to retrieve them. The magic bullet to avoid this is a GnRH analogue, which your doctor includes in your stimulation cocktail. The GnRH analogue blocks your own GnRH and stops you from ovulating. Two types of GnRH analogues can be used:

✔ **GnRH agonists:** Most IVF doctors prescribe an agonist (activator), which you take daily throughout the whole stimulation phase either as a nasal spray or an injection.

✔ **GnRH antagonists:** Antagonists (blockers) have a slightly different action to agonists, are a bit more expensive and are taken as a daily injection only during the last few days of the stimulation phase.

You may experience the following side effects while taking a GnRH analogue:

✔ Headaches

✔ Hot flushes (agonists only)

✔ Irritation at the injection site

✔ Mood swings (agonists only)

✔ Nausea (antagonists only)

GnRH analogues aren't subsidised by Medicare so you pay the full cost of the drug. The clinic may supply you with the drug and then bill you, or you may be given a prescription to fill at a pharmacy.

Human chorionic gonadotrophin

In a normal menstrual cycle a surge in luteinising hormone triggers the final maturation of the eggs and initiates ovulation. Synthetically produced luteinising hormone is available but very expensive. Human chorionic gonadotrophin (hCG) hormone does the same job as luteinising hormone, and so this is used to mature the eggs before egg collection. You have a single injection of hCG about 34 to 37 hours before your eggs are retrieved. Depending on the clinic you may be given synthetically produced hCG or hCG derived from pregnant women's urine.

hCG also works to maintain progesterone levels after embryo transfer, preventing your period from starting before the embryo has a chance to implant. Women who have few follicles sometimes have three doses of hCG instead of receiving progesterone to ensure adaquate progesterone levels (see Chapter 5).

Side effects from hCG are very rare but the following have been reported:

✔ Breast tenderness

✔ Fatigue

✔ Fluid retention

✔ Headaches

✔ Irritability

✔ Irritation at the injection site

hCG is provided for free under Medicare's PBS.

Progesterone

Progesterone is the most important hormone in the second part of the menstrual cycle, the *luteal phase*. This hormone perfects the environment in the uterus for the little embryo to implant and stops a period from starting before the embryo has had a chance to 'stick'.

In IVF treatment you often receive progesterone for a couple of weeks after embryo transfer to make sure that enough of the hormone is in your body to do its job. You take the progesterone in the form of vaginal pessaries or gel, or injections.

Side effects from progesterone are rare but if you use pessaries or gel you may experience vaginal irritation and some discharge.

Progesterone pessaries are small, oval-shaped wax 'pellets' that you insert into your vagina once or twice per day. Your body temperature makes the pellets melt and, while the progesterone hormone is absorbed, the wax turns into a white discharge. So be ready to go through a bundle of panty liners.

Your doctor gives you a prescription for the type of progesterone that you need. Progesterone gel is provided for free on the PBS, but only for stimulated cycles. If you need progesterone after embryo transfer (see Chapter 5), you have to pay for the type of progesterone that your doctor prescribes.

Clomiphene citrate

Clomiphene citrate (CC) is a synthetic anti-oestrogen that tricks the body into thinking that oestrogen levels are low. The body then increases production of FSH, which in turn stimulates follicle growth in the ovaries. For women who don't respond very well to other forms of ovarian stimulation, a course of CC tablets can sometimes yield a few eggs. The tablets are usually taken for five days, starting in the first few days of a cycle.

Possible side effects of CC are usually mild and include

- Blurred vision (let your doctor know if this happens)
- Feeling bloated
- Hot flushes

Your doctor gives you a prescription for CC, which you fill at a pharmacy, and explains when to start taking the tablets and how many to take every day.

Since CC tries to increase your production of FSH, and GnRH analogues shut down FSH and LH production, CC doesn't work together with GnRH analogues. Therefore, if you take CC there's a slight risk that your body may ovulate before your eggs are retrieved. To avoid this happening, when the follicles reach a certain size you undergo daily blood tests to check on the level of luteinising hormone. If the level stays low, egg retrieval is timed with an injection of hCG when the follicle size indicates that the eggs are ready for retrieval. If the level increases and shows that you're getting ready to ovulate, egg retrieval is performed earlier than planned to make sure that the eggs can be recovered.

Estradiol valerate

Estradiol valerate (EV) is a synthetic oestrogen in tablet form that's used to build up the lining in the uterus in preparation for the transfer of frozen embryos. (I talk about frozen embryo transfer in Chapter 5.)

Although side effects of estradiol valerate are rare, you may experience one or more of the following:

- Breast tenderness
- Headaches
- Nausea
- Tummy upset
- Weight gain

Your doctor gives you a prescription for estradiol valerate which you fill at a pharmacy, and explains when to start taking the tablets and how many you need.

Introducing the Common Stimulation Protocols

Not all women follow the same ovarian stimulation protocol: Your protocol depends on your age, your IVF doctor's preference and the clinic's routine.

Figure 6-1 shows a sample protocol demonstrating what drugs to take and when. IVF nurses and doctors use the term *cycle day* (cd for short) to tell you when to take the various drugs. The first day of your period is the first day of the cycle, cycle day 1 or cd 1, the second day is cd 2 and so on. The drugs in ovarian stimulation protocols start on different cycle days; your nurse gives you all the instructions you need to complete your protocol.

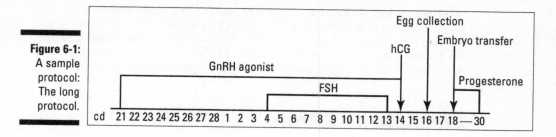

Figure 6-1:
A sample
protocol:
The long
protocol.

In this section I describe the more common stimulation protocols and what they involve.

Long protocol

The *long protocol* is also called the *down-regulation protocol* and — as you probably guess — this protocol takes a while to get through. The reason for this is that you actually start this protocol in the second half of the cycle *before* your planned treatment cycle.

You begin the protocol by taking a GnRH agonist every day, as either an injection or a nasal spray. This drug shuts down your body's own production of follicle-stimulating and luteinising hormones (hence the term *down-regulation*). Such action helps promote the growth of multiple follicles after you start the FSH injections and also stops you from ovulating before the planned egg collection. After a couple of weeks you start FSH injections and these continue until the largest follicles measure at least 18 mm in diameter, after which you have a single injection of hCG to trigger maturation of the eggs ready for retrieval.

Short protocol

In the *short protocol* you start FSH injections on cycle day 2 or 3 and after the follicles reach a certain size you start a GnRH antagonist to stop you from ovulating. After two to five days of receiving the GnRH antagonist you have a single injection of hCG to trigger maturation of the eggs; your eggs are then retrieved two days later.

Flare protocol

During the first couple of days of taking GnRH agonists they cause a flare of follicle-stimulating and luteinising hormones to be released from the brain, but afterwards these hormones are inhibited by the GnRH. The *flare protocol* takes advantage of this temporary increase in FSH, which helps many little follicles to start their growth from the very start of the cycle. After the follicles have started to grow the FSH injections keep them growing; when the largest follicles reach at least 18 mm in diameter you have a single injection of hCG to trigger maturation of the eggs ready for retrieval.

Clomiphene citrate

If you don't respond well to other stimulation protocols, a course of clomiphene citrate (to which your doctor may add FSH injections) can stimulate growth of a few follicles. You usually take CC for five consecutive days, starting early in the cycle. When the largest follicle reaches about 16 mm in diameter, your blood is tested daily to check the level of luteinising hormone and ensure that you aren't about to ovulate before the eggs are retrieved. All being well, the level indicates that you aren't about to ovulate and you have a single injection of hCG to trigger maturation of the eggs ready for retrieval two days later. If the level shows that you're getting ready to ovulate, egg retrieval is brought forward accordingly. Sometimes your doctor prescribes you a GnRH antagonist for the last day or two before the hCG trigger injection, to make sure that you don't ovulate before egg collection.

Going natural

Some women prefer to use the one egg that they ovulate naturally every month rather than having hormone stimulation to produce multiple eggs. Their reason may be that they've suffered bad side effects from the drugs before or have tried various stimulations without success.

If you opt to go natural, you'll have ultrasound and blood tests to try to pinpoint the optimum time for egg collection. Performing natural cycle IVF is very tricky because there's no margin for error: If the one and only egg ovulates before egg collection or is lost during egg collection, you go right back to square one.

Perfecting Your Stimulation Protocol

Certain ovarian stimulation protocols work better for some women than others. Generally speaking, the protocols that include GnRH agonists to prevent ovulation are more commonly used than those that rely on GnRH antagonists (I explain the difference between GnRH agonists and antagonists in the section 'Understanding What Drugs Are Used, and Why' earlier in this chapter). Your doctor discusses your protocol with you: If you don't understand something or want to understand better, just ask your doctor or nurse to explain.

Deciding on your dosage of FSH

The dose of GnRH analogues is the same for all women and stays the same right through the treatment, but the dose of FSH varies for each woman. Your doctor has no way of knowing exactly how you'll respond to FSH when you have your first IVF cycle, but the following criteria can guide the decision regarding the dose of FSH most likely to result in you producing about a dozen eggs:

- ✔ **The number of follicles in your ovaries before stimulation starts:** A vaginal ultrasound of the ovaries shows the number of follicles already there. If you have heaps of little follicles waiting to be stimulated your doctor very cautiously gives you a low dose of FSH, because you could be at risk of developing ovarian hyperstimulation syndrome (an extreme response to the drug, which I explain in Chapter 10).

- ✔ **Your age:** As women get older their response to FSH decreases, so if you're over 38 years of age, you may receive a higher dose of the hormone than if you're younger than 38.

- ✔ **Your response to any previous stimulation attempt(s):** If you've had previous cycles, your doctor checks your previous dosage and how you responded.

- ✔ **Your baseline FSH level:** Your doctor may check the level of FSH present in your blood early in your menstrual cycle to help decide the FSH dose to use.

The daily FSH dose that doctors prescribe ranges from 75 international units (IU) to up to 450 IU.

The most common FSH starting dose for IVF is 150 IU per day. If this dose doesn't result in a sufficient number of eggs, your doctor increases the dose next time. Most doctors won't increase the daily dose beyond 450 IU because for the majority of women this higher dosage doesn't actually help produce any more eggs.

Most doctors err on the side of caution when working out your dose in order not to put you at risk of an over-response, which can cause ovarian hyperstimulation syndrome (I explain OHSS in Chapter 10). If your first cycle is unsuccessful and you decide to try again, your doctor adjusts the dose up or down as determined by your response, in the hope of improving the outcome of the stimulation in the next cycle.

Measuring your response to FSH

After having FSH injections for a week or so you have a vaginal ultrasound scan to check on your response to the drug. The ultrasonographer counts the number of follicles and measures their sizes (I talk more about this examination in Chapter 5). You may also have blood tests to determine your estradiol levels, which is another gauge of your response to ovarian stimulation.

Ideal response

Ideally, the stimulation results in the simultaneous growth of between ten and 15 follicles that reach a size of 18 mm or more in diameter before the final maturation of the eggs is triggered with an hCG injection.

After follicles start growing, they grow by about 2 mm every day. If the scan shows that you have a good number of follicles but they haven't yet reached their optimum size, you're advised to take FSH for another few days before having the hCG trigger injection. Figure 6-2 shows an ultrasound image of an ovary with multiple large follicles (the black holes): An ideal response to IVF stimulation.

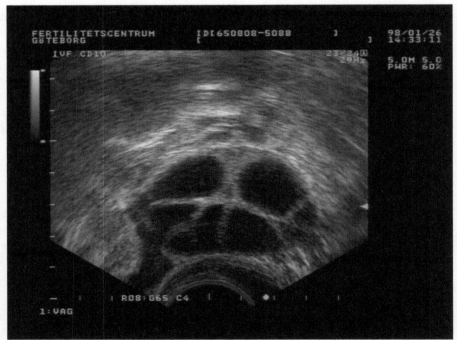

Figure 6-2:
An ideal response to FSH.

The number of follicles you have isn't always an indication of how many eggs you'll get. If you have a couple of large follicles and lots of tiny ones, probably only the larger follicles will produce mature eggs. Even if eggs are found in some of the small follicles, these eggs are unlikely to be mature and able to fertilise.

Not quite enough of a response

Sometimes the result of the stimulation is disappointing. When only one or two large follicles are seen, your doctor may suggest that you stop the treatment and try again with a higher dose. If you're already taking the highest dose, your doctor will probably suggest that you keep going and cross your fingers that one of the eggs is a winner. Figure 6-3 shows an ultrasound image of an ovary where there are only two decent-looking follicles: A disappointing stimulation result.

When the scan shows that you have some small follicles but no large ones, your doctor may increase the dose of FSH and ask you to have another scan a few days later. If the follicles respond to the higher dose, you'll have an hCG injection when they reach the desired size ready for egg collection two days later.

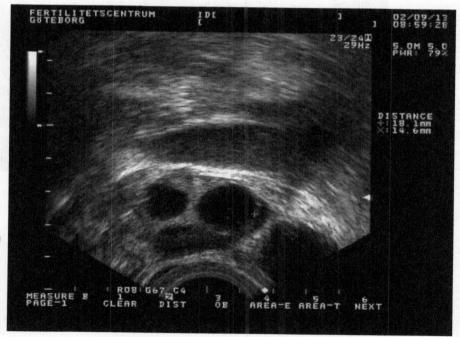

Figure 6-3: A disappointing response to FSH.

Over-the-top response

A very small number of women develop a total over-the-top response to FSH and their ovaries become much enlarged because they're full of growing follicles. In Figure 6-4 you can see what that looks like on ultrasound: Masses of follicles of all sizes crowding the entire ovary. This response is known as ovarian hyperstimulation syndrome and it's every IVF doctor's fear because of the potential danger for the woman. However, managed well the risk can be minimised, and in Chapter 10 I explain what your doctor does to limit your risks.

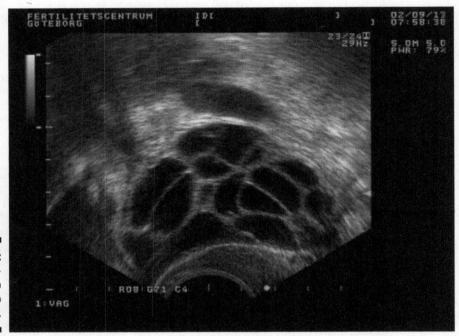

Figure 6-4:
An over-
the-top
response to
FSH.

Chapter 7

Taking a Peek Inside the Lab

The most important part of the IVF process happens behind closed doors in the lab, where a bunch of extremely dedicated and highly skilled embryologists work to make your dream of having a baby come true. The IVF lab is a place with strict rules: The embryologists follow detailed protocols and rigorous quality control measures to provide the ideal environment for eggs and sperm to develop into healthy embryos and to guarantee foolproof systems for keeping track of which eggs, sperm and embryos belong to you.

In this chapter, I take you inside the lab and show you how embryologists give nature a helping hand. I also explain how embryologists help you to boost your chances of IVF success by freezing some of your embryos.

Getting Ready for You

The embryologists are involved in the management of your treatment. They review your medical history close to egg collection and make sure that they're ready to take good care of the eggs and sperm when they're delivered to the lab. The following information helps the embryologists to estimate how many eggs you'll have and what your sperm quality may be like, in order to adequately prepare for your treatment:

- ✔ Any special treatments requested by your doctor
- ✔ Cause of your infertility
- ✔ Number of follicles seen on ultrasound
- ✔ Results of any previous treatment cycle(s)
- ✔ Sperm test results (refer to Chapter 1)
- ✔ Your age
- ✔ Your hormone levels
- ✔ Your stimulation protocol (refer to Chapter 6)

The embryologists also check that you've signed all the necessary consent forms, including giving permission for any special procedures that may be needed such as ICSI and embryo freezing.

Labelling Dishes (And Avoiding Mix-Ups)

The embryologists carefully label, check and recheck all the items of equipment that house your eggs, sperm and embryos to make sure that there's no possibility of mix-ups and you don't end up with the wrong embryos. Couples sometimes worry about mix-ups, but you can rest assured that the systems in place in Australian IVF labs to avoid mix-ups are extremely stringent.

Australian IVF clinics have to follow the Reproductive Technology Accreditation Committee's Code of Practice in order to be licensed (you can read more about these licensing requirements in Chapter 4). This code states that:

> *The organisation shall ensure that gametes, embryos and patients are correctly identified and matched at all times.*

That's why the clinic staff check your name and date of birth *over and over again* at every step of the treatment process. Although your doctor and other staff know very well who you are, such name checking and double-checking is extremely important to avoid mix-ups.

Mix-ups and the media

Occasionally you see reports in the media of mix-ups in IVF labs. Mostly these mix-ups happen because staff fail to follow basic procedures like checking a woman's name before transferring the embryos. Several such cases have made the headlines in recent years:

- In the United States a woman gave birth to a little boy who subsequently turned out to be the genetic child of another couple who attended the clinic at the same time.

- In the United Kingdom a white couple and a black couple were treated in a clinic at the same time. The white woman subsequently gave birth to mixed-race twins and genetic testing showed that while she was

their biological mother, her eggs had been fertilised incorrectly with sperm from the black man.

- A young Japanese woman was mistakenly implanted with the embryo of a 40-year-old woman. The young woman became pregnant but had to have an abortion because the foetus didn't develop properly and it was then revealed that the wrong embryo had been transferred.

Events like these are certainly tragic, but you need to put them in perspective: Of the millions of IVF cycles performed worldwide every year, a mix-up is a rare event, occurring only once every couple of years or so.

Preparing Your Eggs and Sperm

Before your eggs and sperm can finally meet, the embryologist has to prepare them to maximise the chances of a successful union. Eggs need to be perfectly mature and sperm 'cleaned up' before the two are introduced: Embryologists are meticulous in doing everything they can to facilitate the process of fertilisation and embryo development.

Checking your eggs

Immediately after egg collection, the embryologist places your eggs in a special dish with culture medium — fluid specifically made for eggs — and puts the dish in an incubator. The environment in the incubator is regulated so that the temperature, gas and pH levels are the same as in a woman's body — this ensures that the eggs feel 'at home'.

The embryologist can then take a closer look at the eggs and record the fine detail about each egg. The embryologist is hoping to find eggs that are 'just right', as they have the best chance of fertilising. In 'just right' eggs, the embryologist can see that a polar body has been extruded, which means that the egg has rid itself of half its original 46 chromosomes in preparation for the 23 chromosomes that the sperm brings. 'Just right' eggs are also surrounded by a fluffy cloud of so-called cumulus cells, which nourish the egg. The more eggs that are 'just right', the happier the embryologist.

The look of the eggs and the surrounding cells determines how long the embryologist needs to wait before introducing them to the sperm. This is called the *pre-incubation time* and it can range from one hour to several hours. For ICSI, the embryologist removes all the cells surrounding the eggs before injecting the sperm and this allows a detailed assessment of the maturity of the eggs.

If the cells surrounding the eggs appear very tightly packed, the eggs may be immature. The embryologist gives potentially immature eggs a long pre-incubation time in the hope that this will allow the eggs to progress through the maturation process. Although this improves their chance of fertilising, such eggs have a lower chance of developing into healthy embryos.

Prepping your sperm

After the embryologist has checked your eggs, he or she moves on to your sperm sample, which in most cases is produced on the day of egg collection (refer to Chapter 5). Sperm need a bit of cleaning up and sorting before they are added to the eggs.

Washing the sperm

The ejaculate consists of sperm mixed in secretions from the seminal vesicles and the prostate called seminal plasma, as well as white blood cells, dead sperm and other 'debris'. The live sperm need to be separated out from this other material before they can be added to the eggs. To do this the embryologist places a layer of special culture medium over the sperm sample. The motile sperm are able to swim through this layer, leaving behind the unwanted material at the bottom of the container. The embryologist then skims the motile, cleaned sperm off the top.

Taking the sperm for a spin

After the motile sperm have been removed they are diluted with culture medium, placed in a test tube and centrifuged (spun) by machine. As they are spun, the best sperm gather as a pellet at the bottom of the test tube. This pellet is harvested and the process is repeated. The end result is a small volume of fluid with a high concentration of motile sperm, perfect for the waiting eggs.

Dealing with hard-to-get sperm

If you have a male factor infertility problem, you'll probably have the intracytoplasmic sperm injection (ICSI) procedure rather than IVF. Sperm preparation techniques for ICSI vary depending on what kind of problem you have and whether sperm are in the ejaculate or surgically retrieved from the testicles. (I explain the different ways of retrieving sperm from the testicles in Chapter 5.)

Developing the Embryos

After the embryologist has completed all the preparatory work, it's time to introduce your eggs and sperm to each other, the aim being to develop embryos. To help things along, the embryologist ensures that the environment is perfect for developing embryos to thrive.

One egg + thousands of sperm = IVF

If you're having IVF, the embryologist adds a droplet of the prepared fluid containing thousands of keen little sperm to each egg. Then the race is on: Only one of the thousands of sperm in each droplet will get the chance to enter the egg's inner sanctum. Many other sperm will attach to the surface of the egg and keep knocking on the door, without being let in, because after the first sperm enters the egg it triggers a chemical reaction that effectively locks the door behind it.

One egg + one sperm = ICSI

If you're undergoing ICSI, the embryologist gives the sperm a helping hand to enter the egg. Since it takes only one sperm to fertilise an egg, the embryologist catches a single sperm and injects it directly into the centre of an egg. If you have several eggs, the embryologist repeats the process.

ICSI sounds simple but is actually a very technically advanced procedure that requires complex equipment and a highly skilled operator. To perform the procedure, the embryologist uses a specialised piece of equipment called a *micromanipulator*, which has two 'arms' — one arm has a specially designed holding pipette (which has a slight suction applied to it) to hold onto the egg; and the other arm has an extremely thin, sharp and hollow needle attached to it to pick up and inject the sperm into the egg. The embryologist delicately steers the 'arms' using knobs and levers.

This is how the procedure works (see also Figure 7-1):

1. Using one of the micromanipulator's 'arms', the embryologist holds an egg still with the holding pipette.

2. The embryologist then steers the other micromanipulator 'arm' towards the chosen sperm and 'catches' it with the needle.

3. The embryologist steers the needle towards the surface of the egg and carefully pushes it through the shell of the egg into the centre of the egg, called the cytoplasm.

4. When the needle is in place, the sperm is injected into the cytoplasm.

5. The embryologist carefully removes the needle and returns the injected egg to the incubator.

These steps are repeated for all the eggs.

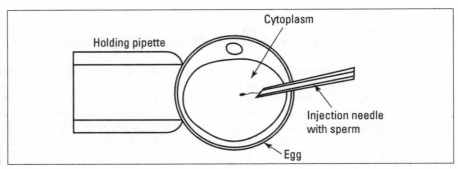

Figure 7-1: Intracytoplasmic sperm injection.

Optimising the environment

Over the next few days the newly introduced eggs and sperm are kept in dishes with culture medium in the incubator where hopefully embryos form during this time. The culture medium and the environment in the incubator closely mimic the conditions in the female body to give the embryos the best chance to form and develop. Embryos don't like changes in temperature or pH levels, so the embryologist makes sure that the eggs and sperm are removed only when absolutely necessary to check on progress and then for as short a time as possible.

Checking on progress

The morning after egg collection the embryologist checks the eggs carefully under a microscope for signs of fertilisation. The embryologist hopes to see two *pronuclei* (PN) inside each egg — one containing the genetic material from the egg and the other containing material from the sperm — because this indicates that the egg has been fertilised normally. About 5 per cent of fertilised eggs are abnormal, in most cases because more than one sperm has been 'let in' so that there are three or more pronuclei instead of two. Figure 7-2 shows a normally fertilised egg with its zona pellucida (egg shell), polar bodies (the material that the egg gets rid of as part of the maturation process in preparation for the 23 chromosomes that the sperm brings) and its two pronuclei (a 2PN embryo).

In some clinics the embryologists check the eggs a second time the day after egg collection to assess the speed of early embryo development, as this gives them an idea of the embryos' potential to develop into an ongoing pregnancy.

On day two after egg collection the embryologist checks the eggs again under the microscope. By now the eggs should have started to divide and form cleavage stage embryos (see the sidebar 'Embryo development'). The embryologist studies each embryo's in detail, looking for the following:

- ✔ **Fragmentation:** Sometimes bits of an embryo's blastomeres break off and cause embryo fragmentation (broken pieces in the embryo). The less fragmentation the better, but only about 20 per cent of embryos have no fragments whatsoever.

- ✔ **Number of blastomeres:** On day two after egg collection the embryo should have three to six blastomeres.

- ✔ **Shape of blastomeres:** The blastomeres should have a spherical shape.

- ✔ **Size of blastomeres:** Ideally, the blastomeres should be of even size.

- ✔ **Zona pellucida (egg shell):** This should be intact with no 'cracks'.

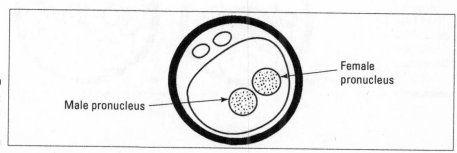

Figure 7-2:
A 2PN
embryo.

Female pronucleus

Male pronucleus

Embryo development

Embryos develop by cell division. Initially, the egg and sperm form a single cell, which has the genetic material of the mother and the father. This cell divides and forms two identical cells. These two cells then divide to form four cells and so on. The early embryo is called a *cleavage stage embryo* and the cells are called *blastomeres*. The daily increase in the number of blastomeres indicates how healthy the embryo is: Three days after egg collection an embryo is expected to have between six and 12 blastomeres. Depending on the clinic's practice, one or two of your embryos are transferred to your uterus two to five days after egg collection.

The embryologist grades the embryos according to their looks. The grading scheme describes the quality of the embryos and their potential to continue to develop after embryo transfer. Information about the quality of the embryos that are transferred allows your doctor to estimate your chance of pregnancy. Clinics vary in the grading systems they use to classify embryo quality, but the best-quality embryos have the greatest chance of developing into babies. These embryos have the expected number of blastomeres, which are even-sized and spherical in shape, no or very few fragments and an intact zona pellucida. In poor-quality embryos more than half the blastomeres are fragmented, and the blastomeres don't all have the same shape or size. Embryos may also be classified as nonviable, which means that they have no intact cells: Such embryos have no chance of continuing their development. Figure 7-3 shows the difference between a four-cell embryo and a fragmented embryo.

Figure 7-3: The difference between (a) a four-cell embryo and (b) a fragmented embryo.

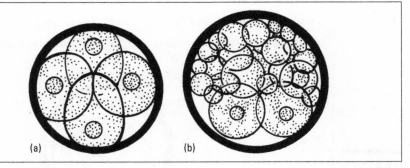

(a)   (b)

Leaving the incubator

Clinics vary in how long they wait before transferring your embryos after egg collection. Some clinics do the transfer two or three days after egg collection, whereas others culture the embryos for five days until they reach the *blastocyst* stage, which is when the embryos have 60 to 100 cells. Most clinics do a bit of both, depending on the number and quality of embryos available. Your doctor can advise about your clinic's policy for timing of embryo transfer and explain the pros and cons of each approach.

Opinions are divided about the best time for embryo transfer:

- Advocates of day two to three transfer argue that the environment in the uterus is superior to even the best lab environment and that an embryo's chance of survival is better the sooner it's transferred to the uterus.

- Supporters of blastocyst transfer believe that by waiting longer you avoid transferring embryos that don't have a really good potential to continue to grow into a healthy baby.

The bottom line is that the number of embryos available for transfer is higher if the transfer is done on day two or three than on day five, but the chance of survival for each individual embryo is lower on day two or three than on day five.

According to the National Perinatal Statistics Unit, which collects and compiles data from all IVF clinics in Australia and New Zealand, blastocyst transfer is gaining in popularity and, in 2006, 27 per cent of all embryo transfers were blastocyst transfers (up from 14 per cent in 2002).

Deciding which embryo to transfer

On the day your embryos are to be transferred, the embryologist assesses all the embryos once more and gives a detailed report about each one to your doctor. When you arrive at the clinic your doctor discusses the report with you and fills you in on what your options are — which of course depend on how many embryos you have and how they've been graded by the embryologist.

If you have more than one embryo ready for transfer, the extras can be frozen and used later. Hopefully, this means you'll get more than one chance to have a baby from the same stimulated cycle.

Hatching help

A procedure called *assisted hatching*, developed in the early 1990s, was hailed as a great advancement in the quest to improve pregnancy rates with IVF. The idea was (and still is) that if the zona pellucida (egg shell) is too tough for the embryo to hatch out of, making a small hole in the zona pellucida could help the embryo. The embryologist makes the microscopic hole using a laser beam or by applying a weak acid solution to an area of the zona pellucida a few hours before embryo transfer.

Although assisted hatching wasn't the great success it was cracked up to be, some clinics still offer the procedure, mainly to older women and to women who've had many embryos transferred unsuccessfully.

Some embryos don't do so well in the incubator and you may find that you have fewer embryos than expected. For example, although you may have had three fertilised eggs the day after egg collection, after two days in the incubator the embryologist may note that two look abnormal in some way or have arrested, meaning that they've stopped developing, and so you have only one embryo ready for transfer.

Putting Your Embryos on Ice

If you agree to embryo freezing and have embryos that are judged good enough for freezing, the freezing process — *embryo cryopreservation* — usually happens on the same day as embryo transfer, although some clinics leave the extra embryos to grow for a bit longer before they freeze them.

The freezing and thawing processes are pretty harsh and only the toughest embryos are candidates for freezing. The embryologist will rate your embryos' chances of getting through such a cold spell. So, even if you have several embryos left over after a stimulated cycle, they may not all qualify for freezing.

Freezing your embryos

The embryos to be frozen are placed in a state of suspense in liquid nitrogen at a cool −196 degrees Centigrade. There are two ways of freezing embryos:

✔ **'Slow freeze' method:** Using this conventional method, the temperature of the embryos is gradually decreased down to the required level. A special chemical is used to protect the cells in the embryo so that damaging ice crystals don't form inside them.

✔ **Vitrification:** Using this newer and faster technique, the embryos are placed in a droplet of a particular solution and then immediately placed in a special container that's cooled by liquid nitrogen. The droplet with the embryo instantly transforms into a glass-like bead. Because the freezing process is so fast, ice crystals don't have enough time to form.

Clinics charge for embryo storage, so if you know you're not going to use embryos that you have stored, you need to notify the clinic about what you want to do with them. Deciding what to do with frozen embryos that you don't plan to use can be very difficult, and I discuss your options in Chapter 15.

Thawing your embryos

If you don't get pregnant after the stimulated cycle and have frozen embryos stored, you can have further embryo transfers without having all the injections required in a stimulated cycle. Frozen embryo transfer is timed so that the lining in the uterus is just right for the embryo to feel welcome and hopefully implant. Your nurse advises you what you need to do when you're ready to have frozen embryos transferred. (I explain when the lining in the uterus is ready for an embryo in Chapter 5.)

The embryologist removes an embryo for thawing and then checks it carefully, recording how it looks compared to when it was first frozen by counting the number of cells, or *blastomeres*, in the thawed embryo: The more intact the embryo, the greater the chance of pregnancy. The embryologist is hoping to find a thawed embryo with all its blastomeres intact, because such embryos are most likely to continue to develop after they're transferred. However, if only a couple of cells have been damaged, an embryo can 'repair' itself. Plenty of healthy children were once embryos that lost a cell or two during freezing or thawing.

The embryos may be thawed the day before the intended transfer date and kept in the incubator overnight or they may be thawed the morning of the day of transfer. If a thawed embryo shows signs of severe damage, another embryo will be thawed out, providing you have more than one embryo stored.

Occasionally, all the frozen embryos in a batch are too damaged to be used. So you may arrive at the clinic ready for embryo transfer only to be told the sad news that no embryos are available because none of the blastomeres has survived. Unfortunately, this means that you have to start another stimulated cycle if you want to try for a baby again.

Chapter 8

Assessing the Odds of Your Dream Coming True

In This Chapter

▶ Understanding the statistics on IVF success rates

▶ Working out your chances of having a baby with IVF

▶ Having realistic expectations

The million-dollar question when you have IVF is: Will the treatment work? There's no way of knowing exactly what your chance of IVF success is, so you have to turn to what's known about IVF success in general to help you estimate your chance of having a baby.

In this chapter, I discuss the issues you need to be aware of when you're looking at how clinics present their results and at IVF statistics in general. I take you through some of the important facts about the odds of getting over the IVF hurdles. I also talk about how you can estimate your own chances of having a baby, considering your circumstances, and how you can try to set realistic expectations and goals.

Getting Over All the Hurdles: What Are Your Odds?

IVF is a series of hurdles that you have to jump over to get what you really want — a baby. At every stage of treatment there's a chance that things may not go according to plan, and each time you make it over one of these hurdles another hurdle looms ahead. In this section I explain what you need to keep in mind when you read clinic statistics about IVF 'success rates' and take you through the 2006 National Perinatal Statistics Unit (NPSU) report, which is the most recent edition of this annual report at the time of writing. The NPSU report outlines the treatment results at each stage of IVF for all clinics in Australia and New Zealand.

The term *success rate* is used to indicate a couple's chance of having a baby with IVF. Sometimes you see this framed as 'successful couples' — which implies that those who don't have a baby after IVF are 'unsuccessful couples'. This terminology is one of my pet hates — there are no unsuccessful couples, only unsuccessful IVF treatments. If treatment doesn't work for you, you're not unsuccessful, just unlucky.

Understanding clinic statistics

To help you assess your chances of success, what you really want to know is, of all the couples who start an IVF treatment cycle, how many have a baby at the end of it? IVF clinics provide various facts and figures about their success rates with couples in general. When you read this information keep in mind that data can be presented in many ways and this presentation can affect your interpretation of the results. Here are a few issues to look out for:

✔ **The denominator used:** Check whether the success rate quoted is a percentage of all couples who:

- Start treatment

- Undergo egg collection

- Have embryo transfer

For example, if out of 100 couples who start IVF treatment 80 undergo egg collection, 70 have embryo transfer and 15 have a baby, the success rate per started cycle is 15 per cent (15 out of 100). However, counted as a percentage of couples who undergo transfer the rate jumps to 21 per cent (15 out of 70) — which sounds much better. Either way, the result is the same: It's just the presentation that differs.

✔ **What counts as success:** Falling pregnant isn't the same thing as having a baby: Not all pregnancies go well. So check whether the success rate quoted refers to all women with:

- A positive pregnancy test

- Clinical signs of pregnancy

- A viable pregnancy confirmed by ultrasound

- A pregnancy beyond 20 weeks

- A live birth

✔ **Who the quoted success rate refers to:** IVF is more successful for some couples than for others, so check whether the quoted success rate is for all couples or for only a selected group that includes couples who have a good prognosis, such as couples:

- Where the woman is younger than 35

- Who don't have complicated infertility problems

- Undergoing their first treatment cycle

Because IVF may not work on your first cycle, it's useful to think about IVF as a series of treatments rather than a one-off treatment. So instead of focusing on what your chance may be if you have just one cycle without any additional transfers of frozen embryos, ask your doctor to give you an idea of how likely you are to have a baby if you were to have three stimulated cycles, including transfer of frozen embryos from these stimulated cycles. Depending on your personal circumstances, your chance may be as high as 75 per cent.

Interpreting the NPSU report

When you're trying to get your head around the NPSU's IVF statistics, it's important to remember that the data reflect the *average* of what happens to *all* couples undergoing IVF treatment. The data include the young and the old, couples on their first treatment cycle and those on their tenth cycle, couples who have lots of eggs and those who have only a few and so on. The report thus provides a *global view* of the workings of IVF.

Note: All statistics in the following sections relate to the year 2006 in Australia and New Zealand.

In 2006 the average live birth rate after a stimulated cycle for all clinics in Australia and New Zealand was 19.6 per cent. Live birth rates vary between clinics, so you may want to look closely at these figures before choosing your clinic (I talk more about choosing a clinic in Chapter 3).

✔ The top 25 per cent of clinics had a live birth rate of 23 per cent or more.

✔ The middle 50 per cent of clinics had a live birth rate between 15.6 per cent and 22.9 per cent.

✔ The bottom 25 per cent of clinics had a live birth rate of 15.5 per cent or lower.

Getting to egg collection

Almost 30,000 stimulated cycles were started, but 10 per cent were cancelled before egg collection. The most common reasons why cycles are discontinued at this stage are

- Too few large follicles are visible on ultrasound
- Hormone levels indicate that the best time for egg collection has passed
- Too many follicles are seen on ultrasound or hormone levels indicate an excessive response to stimulation (I explain the risk of ovarian hyperstimulation syndrome in Chapter 10.)
- Ultrasound picks up a cyst or some other problem that needs to be fixed before egg collection

Of the women who underwent egg collection, about 1.5 per cent had the misfortune of not getting any eggs.

Reaching the embryo transfer stage

Of all the women who had eggs collected, 88.5 per cent had an embryo transfer. The common reasons why some couples don't get to embryo transfer include

- None of the eggs fertilise
- The eggs don't fertilise normally and so can't be transferred
- The fertilised eggs arrest, meaning that they fertilise normally and may even start to divide but then stop developing
- The woman's high risk of ovarian hyperstimulation syndrome means the safest option is to freeze the embryos and wait for her hormone levels to settle down before transferring one or two of the frozen embryos (I explain why this is a safer option in Chapter 10.)

Falling pregnant

The NPSU report uses the term *clinical pregnancy* to define pregnancy and it includes

- Ectopic pregnancies (when the embryo implants and starts to grow in the fallopian tube or somewhere else outside the uterus)
- Miscarriages
- Pregnancies where a sac with a foetus can be seen on ultrasound inside the uterus; the foetus may or may not have a heartbeat
- Pregnancies that are still going at 20 weeks gestation

Of the couples who started stimulated cycles, 25.2 per cent had a clinical pregnancy; and of the couples who reached embryo transfer, 32.1 per cent had a clinical pregnancy.

Having a baby

Aha, the most important statistic:

- ✔ 19.6 per cent of couples who started a stimulated cycle had a live birth
- ✔ 25 per cent of couples who had an embryo transfer had a live birth

So, one in five couples who started a stimulated cycle had a baby and these odds improved to one in four for those couples who reached the embryo transfer stage.

Increasing the odds with embryos on ice

Of the approximately 17,500 cycles that were started with the intention of transferring frozen embryos, almost 91 per cent resulted in an embryo transfer and the remainder were discontinued because none of the embryos survived. Of the couples who had a transfer, 20.7 per cent had a clinical pregnancy and 15.5 per cent had a live birth.

Understanding Your Chances of IVF Success

So, what are *your* odds of having a baby with IVF? The answer is: It depends. Several factors are at work here:

- ✔ Factors relating to you as a couple, such as your age, the cause of your infertility and lifestyle factors such as being overweight and smoking
- ✔ Factors relating to your treatment, such as what type of treatment you have, how you respond to hormone stimulation, how many eggs are recovered, the number and quality of the embryos, and whether you have frozen embryos

In this section I show how some of these factors play out in the big IVF lottery.

Age

The most important factor that influences your chances of having a baby with IVF is something you can't do anything about: Your age. Most available research shows the negative effect of a woman's age on IVF success, but some evidence now also suggests that the male partner's age negatively affects IVF success.

Table 8-1 includes data from the 2006 NPSU report, which convincingly show that age affects the outcome of IVF. For example, the live birth rate per started cycle is 28 per cent for women in the 30–34 age bracket, but this falls to just 7 per cent for women in the 40–44 age bracket. Even more sobering is the fact that of the 61 per cent of women who reach the stage of embryo transfer in the 45 and over age bracket, less than one per cent have a baby. The figures shown in Table 8-1 are for couples who used the female partner's eggs; older women who use eggs donated by younger women fare much better (I talk about egg and embryo donation in Chapter 13).

Table 8-1	The Effect of a Woman's Age on IVF Outcomes		
Age	*Embryo Transfer*	*Clinical Pregnancy per Started Cycle*	*Live Birth per Started Cycle*
24 or less	71%	33%	28%
25–29	80%	34%	28%
30–34	82%	33%	28%
35–39	80%	25%	19%
40–44	72%	12%	7%
45 or over	61%	2%	0.7%

Stimulation response

The more eggs you get, the greater your chances of having a baby with IVF. Although age is the most important factor affecting the number of follicles that develop and the number of eggs you get, the fact is some women respond well to hormone stimulation and others don't, and these differences aren't just age-related. For example, some women in their late thirties get 20 eggs while some women in their late twenties struggle to get a few eggs.

If you get only a few eggs in a stimulated cycle, your doctor will usually increase your dose of follicle-stimulating hormone (FSH) if you try another cycle (refer to Chapter 6). This increase in FSH may increase the number of eggs you get, but only to a point. In most cases your response to FSH tends to stay within a certain range, so if you get three eggs on the first cycle and the dose of FSH is increased on the second cycle, you may get six eggs but you're unlikely to get, say, 15 or 20. Likewise, if you respond well in the first cycle and have the same dose of FSH in subsequent cycles, you're likely to respond well again each time.

Type of fertility problem

Your chance of having a baby varies slightly depending on the type of infertility you have.

- **Male factor infertility:** Couples with male factor infertility have the best odds of having a baby with IVF technology and in 2006 had a live birth rate of almost 22 per cent per started stimulated cycle and almost 17 per cent per frozen embryo transfer.

- **Female factor infertility:** Couples with female factor infertility have slightly lower odds of having a baby with IVF technology and in 2006 had a live birth rate of just over 17 per cent per started stimulated cycle and just over 14 per cent per frozen embryo transfer.

Lifestyle factors

In Chapter 3 I talk about the negative effects of lifestyle factors such as being overweight, drinking alcohol and smoking on fertility in general and on IVF outcomes in particular. Each of these factors reduces your chances of having a baby by a few percentage points, which is bad seeing the odds can be pretty low anyway. But if all these factors are combined, that really leaves you with very little chance of achieving your dream.

Changing your lifestyle may be hard, but to fulfil your dream of having a baby with IVF you need to eliminate as many — and preferably all — of the lifestyle factors that reduce your chances of success *before* you start treatment.

Refer to Chapter 3 for tips on kicking your bad lifestyle habits and improving your general health.

Setting Some Realistic Goals

Of course you're optimistic that IVF will work for you, otherwise you wouldn't start treatment in the first place, and it's important you stay positive and optimistic. But you also need to be realistic.

After you've digested all the information about the odds of getting from A to Z in your IVF treatment program and considered your own particular circumstances, it's time to set some goals. I don't mean deciding now exactly what you're going to do if *x* happens, but you want to think through some issues in advance. The sorts of things you may want to discuss beforehand with your partner and perhaps with your doctor or counsellor are

- What are your chances of having a baby after one stimulated cycle?
- If the first cycle isn't successful, will you try again?
- How many times are you prepared to try?
- How much IVF treatment can you afford? I talk about the costs of treatment in Chapter 3.

Completing your first treatment cycle

Every time you try to conceive with IVF there's a chance the treatment will work. If you're lucky, it may work the very first time for you. In one study of 200 women who were pregnant as a result of IVF, 26 per cent were fortunate enough to conceive on their first go. If it's bingo for you first time, you'll think IVF is pretty easy and that all the talk about how hard it can be to conceive with IVF is nonsense: You have a 100 per cent personal success rate.

If you're unsuccessful on your first attempt to conceive with IVF, you may be encouraged to know that in the same study of 200 women, 68 per cent conceived within 12 months of treatment and on average they had 3.5 transfers, including transfers of frozen embryos, before hitting the jackpot.

Trying again

If your first cycle is unsuccessful and you don't have frozen embryos or have used your frozen embryos, you're back at square one and you have to decide whether you can face another treatment cycle.

Some couples take time out after an unsuccessful cycle and think long and hard about whether or not to try again. Others feel better if they just keep going and are ready to start another cycle as soon as they get the go ahead from their doctor. For yet others the experience of a failed IVF cycle is more than they can take and they decide not to try again.

Most couples pick up the courage to start another cycle and some persist until they get the desired outcome, even if they have to try many times. You have to work out how you feel and agree with your partner if and when to start again.

Two of your IVF team in particular can help you with your decision:

✔ Your counsellor can help you consider the pros and cons and provide you with some coping strategies and survival tips before you embark on another cycle.

✔ Your doctor will use the information from your first cycle to try to improve your chances if you try again and can perhaps shed some light on why things didn't go to plan. You may like to ask your doctor about the following:

- Are there any clues as to why the cycle didn't work?

- Were the number and quality of eggs satisfactory? Can the stimulation be modified to get more or 'better' eggs next time?

- Was the number of eggs that fertilised satisfactory? If not, are there ways to try to increase the number next time, perhaps by using ICSI if you didn't have that the first time?

- Was the quality of the embryos satisfactory? If it wasn't, are they likely to be unsatisfactory again?

- Do you need to undergo any tests or procedures before trying again?

If you do decide to try again, ask your doctor how soon you can come back. Some clinics ask you to take a break between cycles, to let your hormone levels settle before starting again.

Chapter 9

Riding the Emotional Roller-Coaster of the IVF Cycle

In This Chapter

▶ Preparing for the roller-coaster by knowing what to expect
▶ Dealing with good news and bad news
▶ Sending out an SOS when things get on top of you

An IVF cycle is often described as an emotional roller-coaster ride during which you sometimes feel hopeful and optimistic and at other times sad and low-spirited. In this chapter, I describe the events that can make your emotions swing during an IVF cycle and give you some strategies for dealing with your feelings and staying in control while you're having treatment. In Chapter 11, I talk more about how the whole infertility and IVF experience can affect your life and sometimes almost drive you round the bend.

Preparing For the Ups and Downs of the IVF Cycle

Researchers around the world have conducted many studies of couples undergoing IVF to get a better understanding of what parts of the treatment they find most distressing. In this section, I give you an idea of the 'pressure points' couples describe through the stages of an IVF cycle. Knowing how others feel during IVF treatment and how they cope can help you prepare for your own IVF journey.

Starting treatment

When embarking on IVF, most couples are glad to be getting on with things and feel good about doing something proactive towards making their baby dream a reality.

However, some couples also report feeling stressed at the start of their treatment. Reasons for stress at this stage vary, but the most common are

- ✔ Being scared of injections and medical procedures
- ✔ Fearing the unknown
- ✔ Feeling overwhelmed with information
- ✔ Feeling nervous about not remembering all the instructions and 'stuffing things up'
- ✔ Worrying about the outcome of treatment

So if you're nervous about starting treatment, you're not alone. You may find talking to a counsellor helpful: counsellors have plenty of experience dealing with worried and nervous couples and can give you some tips for coping at this stage. If you're worried about the medical procedures, remember forewarned is forearmed: Read up as much as you can about the treatment process and ask your doctor or nurse if you're not sure about anything.

Taking drugs and getting all hormonal

Some women really don't like having hormone injections, which is quite understandable. The jabs themselves involve a bit of a 'yuk factor'. Add to this the common side effects of the drugs — feeling bloated and uncomfortable, and having tender breasts, headaches and mood swings — and it's not hard to see why women dislike hormone stimulation.

I talk more about the drugs you take and their side effects in Chapter 6.

Passing the test of egg making

Couples often feel on tenterhooks about finding out on ultrasound how many follicles have developed. The ultrasound scan in a stimulated cycle is a pretty crucial moment in IVF, because the scan tells you a lot about your chances of having a baby. Here's why:

- More follicles = more eggs
- More eggs = more embryos
- More embryos = more transfers
- More transfers = better chance of having a baby

No wonder couples can get a bit anxious and worried at this stage in their cycle.

In Chapter 5 I look at follicle stimulation, including what problems you may encounter at this stage.

Getting eggs and sperm to the lab

The egg collection procedure is a pretty stressful event for most couples. A lot is at stake at this stage of treatment and couples often worry about:

- The procedure itself (the doctor does use a very long needle) and undergoing anaesthetic
- Whether enough eggs will be recovered
- Whether the male partner will be able to produce a sperm sample
- The quality of the sperm sample

For more information on egg collection and the sperm sample see Chapter 5, where I also advise how to cope if you get fewer eggs than expected and/or have a poor sperm sample.

Counting your chickens (or embryos in this case)

Between egg collection and embryo transfer you have plenty of time to worry about how the eggs and sperm will get along and how many embryos you'll get. The number of embryos you get is such an important indicator of how likely you are to have a baby with IVF, so it's hardly surprising that most couples find this wait nerve-racking.

In Chapter 5 I explain what can go wrong at this stage in the cycle and how to pick yourself back up if you end up with no embryos.

Waiting to find out whether the embryo will 'stick'

Not unexpectedly, the majority of couples find the two-week wait between embryo transfer and getting their pregnancy test result very tense. Only two things are perceived as more distressing than this wait — a negative pregnancy test result and losing a pregnancy — which is hardly surprising.

For some tips on getting through this long wait, see Chapter 5.

Taking it like a man

Men can easily become a bit marginalised during IVF treatment because all attention is on the woman — until the crucial moment when the sperm sample is to be delivered and then it's expected pronto! But, of course, whatever ups and downs a woman goes through during the IVF cycle affect her partner too. Naturally, men worry about whether the treatment is going to work, but sometimes they don't show their feelings because they think they need to be strong for their partner.

It's hard for you as a man to see your partner go through the hard yakka of IVF treatment and not be able to do much to help. But your most important contribution to making IVF easier for your partner is to be available throughout treatment, to take time to listen when she wants to talk, and to give her as much love and support as you can.

Feeling High and Feeling Low

As you inch your way through the IVF cycle you get progress reports along the way. If the news is good you'll feel really happy and optimistic about your chances of having a baby. And, of course, if the news is bad you'll be extremely disappointed.

How you feel about your progress reports is affected by what you expect the news to be. It's important, but also difficult, to find the right balance between feeling optimistic about the treatment working and having realistic expectations about the chance of success. I discuss setting realistic goals in Chapter 8.

Feeling on top of the world

IVF is a numbers game and as you play the game you always look at the crucial numbers. These are

- The number of follicles that develop
- The number of eggs recovered
- The number of eggs that fertilise normally and divide
- The number of embryos available for transfer and freezing

And all along it's a case of 'the more, the merrier'. When you get your progress reports, you hope for something like this:

- Your scan shows that you have 12 to 15 large follicles
- Your hormone levels are 'just right'
- You get 12 really mature-looking eggs at egg collection
- Ten of your eggs fertilise normally and start to divide
- You have one perfect-looking embryo ready for transfer
- You have seven other perfect-looking embryos that can be frozen and kept for later

Such reports would make anyone on IVF feel on top of the world. But if you're over 38 years of age or have had a previous unsuccessful cycle with very few follicles and eggs and poor-quality embryos, your expectations will probably be pretty low when you try again. In that case, the following progress reports may make you feel very happy:

- Your scan shows that you have four large follicles
- Your oestradiol level is rising and indicates that the eggs are mature
- You get four eggs at egg collection and they all look great
- Three of your eggs fertilise normally and divide at the expected rate
- You have a beautiful cleavage stage embryo ready for transfer
- The remaining two embryos can be frozen and kept for later

It's fair to say that news about the progress of your IVF cycle is always good if it matches or is better than what you expect.

Discovering that things don't always go to plan

In IVF, bad news can come out of the blue: Sometimes a progress report is much worse than you expect and your dream of a baby seems to float out of reach. The kind of news you hope never to get includes

- ✔ Your scan shows only one or two large follicles
- ✔ Your hormone levels aren't 'right'
- ✔ You have nine large follicles but only two eggs are recovered
- ✔ You have 11 eggs but only two fertilise normally and only one divides
- ✔ You have six embryos but they're all poor quality
- ✔ You have seven embryos but only one is good enough to be transferred and none pass the quality check for freezing

Receiving bad news about your IVF treatment when you don't have your partner with you adds to the injury. Whenever practically possible, make sure that your partner's with you at the clinic if you know you're getting a progress report. If your partner can't be with you, ask someone else you feel close to and trust to attend the clinic with you for moral support.

Treatment sometimes fails; you don't fail

The language used to describe infertility and bad IVF outcomes can make you feel even worse than you already feel, because the terms imply that *you* had something to do with the failure. For example:

- ✔ Your doctor may tell you that you have 'hostile mucus', which could make you wonder how to make it friendlier — as if you could do anything to change it.

- ✔ If you don't develop a lot of follicles after ovarian stimulation you may be called a 'poor responder' — as if you were doing it on purpose.

- ✔ When your eggs don't fertilise or your embryos don't implant, you may be told it's because they were of 'poor quality' — as if you could have done something to produce better quality 'goods'.

- ✔ Couples who have babies after IVF treatment are referred to as 'successful' — which implies that those who don't have babies are failed couples.

Whether IVF works or not is beyond your control and the fact that treatment fails is no reflection on you — it isn't the result of something you have, or haven't, done.

When a progress report is bad news you can easily start worrying whether IVF is ever going to help you to have a baby. After a disappointing cycle you may want to try again but dread the possibility that it'll all be for no gain.

Your doctor and the embryologist review all the information gathered about your hormone stimulation and the quality of your eggs, sperm and embryos to try to pinpoint why things didn't go to plan. Your doctor can advise whether the poor results are likely to happen again or if you were just unlucky. This should help you decide what to do next.

Finding a Helping Hand

The road through an IVF cycle can be rocky and you may need a helping hand here and there along your journey, especially if you undergo several treatment cycles.

Supporting each other

Your greatest supporter is your partner. The two of you have the same goal and have decided to give it your all to have a baby together. However, at times you may both be feeling down and have trouble giving each other support. If that's the case it may be better to turn to someone else for support and focus on nurturing your relationship with your partner instead: Have fun together, go to the movies, eat out, see your friends, go for walks, do anything you like to take a break from the 'IVF job' and to remind yourselves that there's more to your relationship than surviving IVF.

Talking to your team

Make good use of the professionals at your clinic: They're there to help you get pregnant, but also to support you through the IVF process.

Talking to your doctor

Being well-informed about the IVF process and knowing what happens at every stage helps you feel in control and makes you an active participant in your own treatment. Turn to your doctor with any questions you have about your treatment. IVF doctors have a wealth of knowledge and clinical experience and can provide support, guide you through your treatment options, help you evaluate your chances of having a baby, suggest changes to your treatment plan to increase your chances of success and point you to other useful sources of information if you want to know more.

Talking to the nurses

IVF nurses are on top of all the day-to-day information about the progress of your treatment and they 'hold your hand' and give you instructions through a treatment cycle. However, they also understand how stressful IVF can be and are very good at helping you to manage the stress. You can always turn to the nurses with any questions or concerns — if they can't help you, they'll find someone who can.

Talking to the counsellor

If you feel that the stress of IVF is getting to you and no-one understands what you're going through and how you feel, try talking to one of the clinic counsellors. They've seen and heard it all before and can help you get back on top. A session with the clinic counsellor is bound to make you feel better. You can see the counsellor on your own or with your partner — whatever feels right for you. And you may feel better after one session with the counsellor or you may need several sessions, anything is possible.

Calling a friend

If you have a relative or close friend who you think will be willing and available to provide you with support and encouragement while you're on the IVF program, sign 'em up. It's very useful to have someone to turn to and bounce things off who's a bit arm's length from it all but who has your wellbeing at heart.

Part III
Understanding the Risks of IVF

Glenn Lumsden

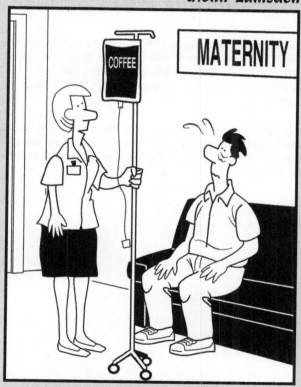

'The twins are doing fine, but the doctor thought you may need this for the next few years.'

In this part . . .

*I*n the hands of experts, IVF procedures are safe and medical complications are rare. But your emotional health can take a beating when you have IVF and sometimes, no matter how hard you try, the treatment doesn't work.

In this part, I explain the potential risks involved with IVF to your physical and mental health and discuss how you can move on and get your life back on track if IVF doesn't work for you.

Chapter 10

Understanding the Risks of IVF to Your Physical Health

In This Chapter

▶ Weighing up the risks involved for the female partner

▶ Checking out the risks involved for the male partner

▶ Considering the health of IVF children

As with all medical procedures, IVF involves some potential risks that you should be aware of before you decide to embark on treatment. You need to consider firstly the risks that relate directly to the IVF procedure and secondly health problems that may develop down the track because you've undergone IVF. But the most burning question for couples who have IVF is whether their child/children will have more medical problems than children conceived spontaneously.

In this chapter, I outline what's known about the possible short- and long-term risks of IVF treatment to the female and male partners, and to the baby.

It's not always possible to say with certainty whether adverse health outcomes found in couples who've undergone IVF are caused by the IVF technique itself, the underlying cause of the infertility or the fact that, on average, couples who have IVF are older when they have children.

Understanding the Possible Risks to Her

Not surprisingly, the female partner faces more risks related to IVF than the male partner. And, of course, being pregnant and giving birth carry their own potential risks for women.

During treatment

Complications requiring hospital admission of the female partner occur in about 1 per cent of all treatment cycles. Just over half of these admissions are due to symptoms of ovarian hyperstimulation syndrome (OHSS) — a potentially serious medical condition — and the rest occur because of surgical complications from egg collection, such as bleeding and infection. Very rarely, in about 1 in 50,000 treatment cycles, serious complications arise from the general anaesthesia given during egg collection.

In Chapter 6 I outline the potential side effects of the drugs you take during IVF treatment. When follicles develop in response to the hormone injections, mild pelvic pain and feeling bloated are common. In most cases the symptoms are fairly minor and ease over time. But occasionally they become severe and some women, especially those who have very large numbers of follicles, develop OHSS. Doctors aren't sure exactly why this happens, but the hormone production associated with the growth of a lot of follicles can shift fluid from the bloodstream into the abdominal cavity and chest. In very rare cases this can lead to blood clots, kidney failure and respiratory problems — even death.

OHSS is categorised depending on the severity of the symptoms:

- **Mild:** Your ovaries are a bit enlarged and you feel bloated and uncomfortable. The pain and discomfort can slow you in your tracks for a few days and you may need to take painkillers. About one in three women get mild OHSS as a result of the IVF hormone stimulation.

- **Moderate:** Your ovaries are enlarged and the pain and discomfort are pretty severe. Your tummy feels really tender and swollen and you may have trouble doing up your pants or skirt. Your doctor may admit you to hospital to keep an eye on things and give you adequate pain relief. About one in 250 women are admitted to hospital with moderate OHSS.

- **Severe:** Your ovaries are several times their normal size, you have a lot of fluid in your abdomen and around your lungs, and you have severe pain. For one in 1,000 women the symptoms of OHSS are so severe that they need treatment in an intensive care unit.

OHSS is self-limiting and in most women the symptoms disappear by the time their next period starts. However, if you're pregnant the symptoms may take a turn for the worse and you may need to be admitted to hospital until things settle down.

Your doctor does several things to reduce the risk of OHSS:

- ✔ Prescribing the lowest possible dose of follicle-stimulating hormone
- ✔ Cancelling your cycle if the ultrasound scan shows that you're growing masses of follicles or your hormone levels are too high
- ✔ Freezing your embryos and deferring embryo transfer to avoid you getting pregnant until your ovaries have returned to normal

You may feel just fine when you leave the clinic after your embryo transfer, but a few days later you may start to get symptoms of OHSS. Mild symptoms occasionally get worse pretty quickly, so contact the nurses or your doctor if you think you're developing OHSS.

Down the track

Like many women on IVF, you may wonder whether the fertility drugs you take to stimulate your ovaries increase your risk of developing cancer some time in the future. The good news is that studies to date haven't found more cases of cancer among women who use fertility drugs than among women in general, and no evidence exists that IVF drugs cause cancer. However, it's only in the last 20 years that IVF drugs have been used by large numbers of women, so doctors still can't be sure that the fertility drugs cause no really long-term health problems.

Pregnancy loss

Unfortunately, even hard-earned IVF pregnancies are sometimes lost. About one in five IVF pregnancies are lost before 20 weeks gestation — a slightly higher rate than after spontaneous conception. There are several possible reasons for this, including the fact that IVF parents are older and more likely to have a multiple pregnancy than other couples. In addition, the underlying cause of a couple's infertility may increase the risk of pregnancy loss.

Pregnancies can be lost in following ways:

- ✔ **Ectopic pregnancy:** Occasionally the embryo implants in one of the fallopian tubes instead of in the uterus. Without intervention, the fallopian tube can burst when the pregnancy grows, causing life-threatening internal bleeding for the woman. Therefore, ectopic pregnancies have to be removed. This can be done surgically or by injecting a drug called methotrexate, which stops the foetus from growing and ends the pregnancy.

You can rest assured that having an ectopic pregnancy doesn't jeopardise your chances of having a pregnancy in the right place if you decide to try IVF again.

IVF pregnancies are monitored closely and the first ultrasound to confirm that the pregnancy is in the right place is undertaken four weeks after embryo transfer. So you're unlikely to experience symptoms caused by an ectopic pregnancy before you have your first scan. But, if you haven't yet had your first scan and experience abdominal or pelvic pain or unexpected bleeding, contact your doctor immediately.

✔ **Miscarriage:** On ultrasound examination your doctor may discover that the foetus is smaller than expected and doesn't have a heartbeat. Or, it may become obvious that you have a so-called *blighted ovum*, which is when the part of the embryo that makes the placenta is growing but the part that is supposed to become the foetus isn't growing.

Sometimes bleeding and cramping signal that you're losing the pregnancy. If you experience such symptoms, contact your doctor immediately.

If you have the misfortune of miscarrying a pregnancy, you're likely to be admitted to hospital for a *dilatation and curettage* (D&C), a minor surgical procedure where the walls of your uterus are scraped to make sure that no tissue is retained from the pregnancy, which can cause bleeding and infection.

✔ **Termination:** In a very small number of cases the foetus has a severe abnormality and you have to make the extremely difficult decision whether to continue with the pregnancy, knowing that the baby may die shortly after birth or be born with a serious disability, or to terminate the pregnancy. Should this happen, counsellors are of course available to help you and your partner through this very distressing time.

Some pregnancy losses happen randomly and others because of factors related to one of the partners, such as a genetic problem. If you have the misfortune of losing a pregnancy after IVF, your doctor will do everything possible to find out why it happened by running all sorts of tests. If anything comes up that gives a clue as to why you lost the pregnancy, your doctor will discuss this with you and if possible tell you whether it's likely to happen again.

Your physical recovery from pregnancy loss is usually uncomplicated, but the sadness and disappointment of being robbed of your dream of having a baby can be very difficult to manage. I talk about the emotional aspects of pregnancy loss after IVF in Chapter 11.

During pregnancy and childbirth

Generally speaking, pregnancy and childbirth are very safe events in countries like Australia with a good healthcare system and most babies are born healthy. But, irrespective of how you conceive, you may have unexpected complications during pregnancy or at the time of birth. Some of these complications are more common with IVF than with spontaneous conception. This is because:

- When more than one embryo is transferred, there's always a chance that you'll have twins (and occasionally triplets) and this is much more risky than a singleton pregnancy.

- Women who have IVF are generally older when they give birth and this increases the risk of pregnancy complications.

Compared with pregnant women in general, women who fall pregnant with IVF are more likely to:

- Be older when they give birth (on average, about five years older)

- Be delivered by caesarean section

- Deliver the baby prematurely

- Have a multiple birth

- Have a baby with lower birth weight

- Have a baby who dies around the time of birth

Pregnancy complications: Facts and figures

When you're considering the risks of pregnancy as a result of IVF treatment, you need to compare these risks with how often complications happen in spontaneously conceived pregnancies. The Australian Institute of Health and Welfare publishes an annual report on Australian mothers and babies. Here are some points to ponder from its latest report:

- 1 in every 6 pregnancies miscarry (1 in 5 after IVF)

- 1 in every 14 babies is born prematurely (1 in 5 after IVF)

- 10 in every 1,000 babies dies around the time of birth (14 in 1,000 after IVF)

- 3 in every 100 babies has some sort of birth defect (6 in 100 after IVF)

Assessing the Possible Risks to Him

As far as health risks resulting from IVF are concerned, the male partner has very little to worry about. However, if you have no sperm in your ejaculate and the sperm has to be obtained directly from your testicles, you do face some minor potential risks.

During treatment

Depending on the nature of your infertility problem, your doctor may perform either a needle biopsy using local anaesthesia to get small pieces of tissue from your testicles or an open biopsy using a general anaesthetic to surgically remove pieces of tissue from your testicles (see Chapter 5) — in both cases so that the embryologist can retrieve sperm from this tissue for ICSI (see Chapter 7). About five to ten out of every 1,000 sperm retrieval procedures result in a complication from either bleeding or infection. The risk of complications is lower for needle biopsy than for open biopsy. In addition, having a general anaesthetic poses a very small health risk.

Down the track

Men who have very low sperm production sometimes have low testosterone levels, and sperm retrieval procedures like testicular biopsy can reduce the production of testosterone even further because some of the testosterone-producing tissue is removed. If you have very low levels of testosterone, you may need testosterone replacement therapy to raise the levels.

Examining the Possible Risks to Baby

'What's the risk of IVF to my baby?' is the most common question asked by couples considering IVF. To date more than two million children have been born as a result of IVF, so doctors have a lot of reliable information with which to answer this question. Mostly the news is good, but there are some adverse outcomes that, rare as they are, are more common among IVF children than children in general. This is often because multiple births are more common with IVF, but it's impossible to exclude the possibility that the IVF technique itself may also contribute to the increased risks.

Some extremely unusual conditions, such as Beckwith-Wiedemann syndrome (BWS), appear to be more common with IVF than with spontaneous conception. Children born with BWS experience overgrowth in certain parts of their body — most commonly the tongue and abdominal wall — and can have very low blood sugar levels and ear abnormalities. An Australian study found that whereas the overall incidence of BWS is one in every 35,000 children born, the risk of BWS with IVF is about four in every 15,000 children born.

Of course, you need to be well informed and understand the risks involved in any medical procedure before going ahead with it, but it's also important to remember that the vast majority of children, including those conceived in a lab through IVF, are born healthy and grow up without any major health problems.

During pregnancy

Women who conceive through IVF have a slightly higher risk of miscarriage and ectopic pregnancy than women who conceive spontaneously. To make sure that everything is going well your doctor refers you for an ultrasound scan very early in your pregnancy, usually four weeks after embryo transfer. If the scan shows a foetus with a heartbeat in your uterus at that early stage, this is a very good prognostic sign and you can allow yourself to relax and feel really happy.

Sometimes you may find out that you're pregnant with twins at your first ultrasound examination only to have one foetus at your next check. There are many reasons for a so-called vanishing twin and there's nothing doctors can do to prevent the loss of one twin.

Childbirth

The Australian Institute of Health and Welfare publishes data about all babies born as a result of IVF in Australia and New Zealand and the organisation's data show that compared with other babies, IVF babies:

- ✔ Are more likely to be a twin
- ✔ Are born after a shorter pregnancy
- ✔ Are more likely to be born prematurely (less than 37 weeks of gestation)
- ✔ Have a slightly higher risk of birth defects and problems like cerebral palsy
- ✔ Weigh slightly less at birth

Many of the added risks for IVF babies are explained by the fact that IVF pregnancies produce many more twins than does spontaneous conception. A good way to avoid some of these risks is to transfer only one embryo. Embryo freezing (see Chapter 7) allows you to play it safe and have one baby at a time rather than putting yourself and your babies at risk.

However, even singleton IVF babies are twice as likely as other babies to be born prematurely and to have a low birth weight. This is thought to be mainly due to IVF mothers being older than other mothers and to IVF parents' underlying fertility problems.

Growing up

Many studies have looked at the health, growth and physical development of IVF children, and most report very few differences between IVF and spontaneously conceived children. Other studies have compared the social, emotional and intellectual development of IVF and spontaneously conceived children and found no differences. So, you have every reason to feel reassured that children born as a result of IVF are as healthy and happy as, and do at least as well as, their peers.

Some people are concerned that children born as a result of IVF may have a higher risk of developing cancer, but this doesn't seem to be the case. Thankfully, cancer in children is very rare and several large studies have concluded that the risk of childhood cancer is the same for IVF children as for other children. Future studies will be able to tell whether particular causes of infertility or forms of infertility treatment increase the risk of childhood cancer.

The longer term health of adolescents and adults born as a result of IVF hasn't been investigated yet, because their numbers are still relatively small. But as more and more IVF children are reaching adulthood, some studies are underway comparing the health and development of IVF and non-IVF adults. Several reports have made mention of IVF-conceived adults becoming parents themselves, but it'll be some time before data are available on whether IVF-conceived adults have more infertility problems than those conceived spontaneously.

If the cause of your infertility is genetic or chromosomal, you may pass on this infertility problem to your children. For example, if you have a severe male factor problem, a small part of your Y chromosome (the chromosome that makes you a man) may be missing — so-called Y chromosome microdeletion. If you have a son, he'll likely have the same microdeletion and need ICSI in the future.

Chapter 11

Realising How IVF Can Affect Your Mental Health

Although IVF doesn't pose a great risk to your physical health (see Chapter 10), the possible risks to your mental health and general wellbeing from IVF are probably greater than from most other medical procedures. As well as your immediate reactions to the ups and downs of each step in the treatment process (which I describe in Chapter 9), IVF impacts on the way you feel about yourself, your partner and your life in general — especially when the treatment doesn't work.

In the last few years numerous researchers have studied the ways in which infertility and infertility treatments affect people's feelings and functioning. Evidence shows that such unexpected and unwelcome life events can shake you up in all sorts of ways. In this chapter, I draw on what's known from the research literature to explain how infertility and having IVF treatment can affect your life and your relationship in the short and longer term.

You can't blame the emotional difficulties that you run into while attending the IVF program — and afterwards — entirely on the IVF procedure itself. The fact that you really want a baby and it's not happening plays a great part, too.

Understanding How IVF Knocks You About Emotionally

Of course, people are different and the way you feel about being infertile and having IVF treatment depends on several factors, such as:

- ✔ **How much support you have:** You can cope more easily with difficult patches in your life if you have a good support network and don't feel that you're alone. If you want to broaden your support network, refer to Chapter 2, where I talk more about finding various sources of support.

- ✔ **How you usually deal with difficult situations:** There are many different ways of tackling problems (none of which are right or wrong), but some ways are better at helping you get through problems than others. I discuss the three broad coping styles for dealing with stressful situations in the section 'Talking about your feelings — often helps her, hinders him' later in the chapter.

- ✔ **Your personality:** Some people are quite robust and seem to be able to take life's challenges on the chin, whereas others are more vulnerable and struggle under pressure.

- ✔ **Your relationship:** If you and your partner support each other and talk openly about how you feel, chances are you'll have fewer emotional problems than if you have trouble communicating with your partner and don't feel loved and cared for. I give you some tips for working together with your partner throughout your IVF journey in Chapter 2.

You may sail through IVF without any difficulties and, if you do, good for you. But if you're like most people, you'll experience some negative feelings from time to time during treatment and when you do it may help you to know that these feelings are normal and that you're not the only one feeling this way.

How you cope emotionally with IVF depends largely on your personal circumstances. It goes without saying that if you're young, start IVF as soon as you find out you have a fertility problem and fall pregnant and have a baby after your first cycle, you'll be far less emotionally affected by the process than if you're 40, have been trying for a baby naturally for ten years, endure six IVF cycles and then suffer a miscarriage.

Realising you may be sad, but you're not mad

Many studies use measures of mood and anxiety to gauge how infertile couples feel throughout their IVF journey. The research clearly shows that keeping your spirits up through the turmoil of IVF is very hard, and couples commonly feel sad and worried while they're on the IVF program. When you feel really sad about something, it's very hard to enjoy anything in life. If you have trouble getting pleasure out of things you normally enjoy, you need to spend time dealing with your feelings and trying to get joy back into your life.

Symptoms of depression and anxiety are perfectly normal reactions to the extraordinary circumstances of requiring complex, demanding and invasive medical procedures to help you to have a baby. So, if you feel down, helpless, miserable, powerless, gloomy, unhappy or distressed — or all of the above — while you're on the IVF program, you're not crazy — you're just trying to get through a massive life challenge. But watch out for the chronic sadness that sometimes sets in and overshadows every aspect of your life. If you can't shake the blues, you need to talk to — yes, you guessed it — a clinic counsellor.

Feeling good for nothing

When you try really hard to achieve something and are unsuccessful, you understandably get frustrated. And if you keep trying and are still unsuccessful, you may start to wonder whether you're doing something wrong or are just no good at whatever you're trying to achieve. This can be the case when you don't get pregnant with IVF. If you try over and over again and the treatment doesn't work, your self-confidence and self-esteem take a beating.

If you're running low on self-confidence and self-esteem, you may start to feel useless and a failure in all sorts of ways, which in turn makes you depressed and feeling even worse. If you get into this vicious cycle where you feel ever more down in the dumps, you need to seek help, because breaking this cycle on your own can be very difficult. Make time to see an IVF counsellor. The counsellors have seen and heard it all before and can help you get back on top of things.

Coping when life's not as fun as it used to be

Enjoying life as much as you normally do can be hard when you're undergoing IVF treatment, especially when the treatment isn't working. The physical and emotional demands of treatment tend to be a bit of a dampener on your spirits. You may feel that your life has lost its gloss and become bleak and gloomy.

As far as possible, try to keep doing the activities you really enjoy while you're on the IVF program — such as playing a sport, reading, seeing friends or going to the movies. These activities give you a sense of normality and are a chance for you to take a break from the strain of life with IVF.

Hanging In There Together

The big life challenges really put relationships to the test. The way you and your partner deal with the stress of your infertility and IVF treatment can make or break your relationship.

✔ **Gaining strength from each other:** Most couples who go down the IVF path have a strong commitment to each other and to their goal of having children together. Studies show that these couples often have better-functioning relationships than average couples and that they perceive each other as their best source of support when they go through the ups and down of treatment. Some reports even show that the rocky road of IVF can bring partners closer together and make their relationship stronger than ever before.

✔ **Drifting apart:** Sometimes the emotional strain of IVF can be too much and partners have trouble being there for each other. This may be because the partners have different ways of dealing with difficulties or because one partner is more committed to having children than the other. As a result, unfortunately a few relationships don't survive the stress of IVF treatment.

Talking about your feelings — often helps her, hinders him

Studies show that among couples who go through IVF treatment, both women and men get the majority of their emotional support from their partner. Mostly this works well, because there's give and take on both sides of the relationship and when one partner feels down the other steps up to the plate, and vice versa. But what happens when both partners feel down and have trouble coping with the demands of IVF? As a general rule — and it's certainly not true for everyone — women feel better having a good talk about what's troubling them and men feel better if they *don't* talk about things.

People manage stressful situations in different ways. The three broad types of coping styles are

- **Avoidance-oriented:** People who tend to use the avoidance-oriented coping style prefer to dodge the stressful situation altogether. If this is you, you feel better if you don't talk about your failed IVF cycle. You do all sorts of things not to think about it, like immersing yourself in work, playing sport or spending time with people who don't know you're having IVF treatment.

- **Emotion-oriented:** People who tend to use the emotion-oriented coping style throw themselves into the feelings that arise from the stressful situation. If this is you, you want to talk at length to your partner and then five of your best friends about how disappointed, upset, sad, frustrated and worried your failed IVF cycle makes you feel.

- **Task-oriented:** Task-oriented people want to deal with a stressful situation head-on. If this is you, you may want to find out exactly what went wrong, searching high and low for information about how to avoid the same thing happening again, straight away making an appointment with your doctor to ask when you can start the next cycle and how your treatment protocol will be changed so that it works better next time.

Some of these coping styles are more commonly used by women and others are more commonly used by men, but there's no right or wrong coping style. However, when partners who get disappointing news use different coping styles to deal with the inevitable stress, they sometimes clash. So, if it helps you to talk about how bad you feel and it helps your partner *not* to talk about how bad he feels, you may have a problem — unless you understand that you're both hurting and just dealing with the issue in different ways.

Dodging the blame game

When things go wrong you may look for someone to blame. The blaming that sometimes happens when IVF fails includes

- ✔ The fertile partner in a couple blames the partner with the fertility problem

- ✔ A woman who had an abortion as a teenager that resulted in an infection and blocked fallopian tubes blames herself

- ✔ A couple blame each other for waiting too long before trying for a family

- ✔ The doctor is blamed for not giving the right stimulation protocol or for not getting enough eggs

- ✔ The embryologist is blamed for the lack of good-quality embryos

Blaming is counterproductive, because you feel worse and the person you blame feels bad. Truth is, most failed IVF cycles are due to either bad luck or biological factors out of your (and everyone else's) control.

If you feel resentful and get caught up in the blame game, talk to one of the clinic counsellors, who can help you turn your negative feelings into something more productive.

Losing a Pregnancy

While you're dealing with the ups and downs of IVF treatment, the goal at the forefront of your mind of course is to get pregnant, and it's very hard to think beyond that. And then when you finally reach that goal the unthinkable sometimes happens: you lose the pregnancy. Or you find out that you're pregnant with twins, but later in the pregnancy you lose one of the twins — a so-called vanishing twin (see Chapter 10). Few things can be more sad and distressing than losing a pregnancy and if this happens to you, you may feel very down and depressed for a long time afterwards. I cover the physical aspects of pregnancy loss in Chapter 10 and in this section I discuss how you may feel after a pregnancy loss.

Pregnancy loss is a devastating experience, no matter how or why it happens. After the initial shock you're likely to feel very sad for a long time. The earlier in the pregnancy you experience your loss, the quicker people expect you to get over it and move on. But life doesn't quite work like that. Even if you're pregnant for only a few weeks, the grief of losing a pregnancy can be very intense. Your feelings are real and shouldn't be ignored. Seek out the clinic counsellor if you struggle with your emotions after pregnancy loss.

You may even start to think that you did something to cause the loss. Self-blame is common among women who experience pregnancy loss, but the truth is that these things happen for reasons that are totally out of your control. In most cases a pregnancy ends because the foetus doesn't have the right number of chromosomes or has some other abnormality that's incompatible with life. If you decide to try again for a baby, you may feel very anxious that the same thing will happen all over again.

If you find that your worries about repeated pregnancy loss are getting out of hand or if you keep wondering whether you could have done something to prevent your loss, talk to an IVF counsellor. The counsellor can help you to find strategies to manage your anxiety. He or she can also arrange to see you regularly during the early months of a subsequent pregnancy as you wait to find out whether everything is okay.

Sometimes people try to make you feel better after you lose a pregnancy by saying that if there was something wrong with the baby, maybe it was all for the best that you miscarried. Or if you lose one of your twins, well-intended people may tell you that you're lucky one baby is still growing. Comments like these are little comfort and don't stop you wishing that the baby had been healthy or that you hadn't lost one of your twins.

If you lose a pregnancy, it can be tempting to want to get pregnant again as soon as possible to get away from the haunting thoughts of the baby you've just lost. But it's important to allow yourself time to grieve your loss. The grieving process allows you to heal and move on, even if you still feel sad when you think about the loss.

The grieving process after pregnancy loss can be hindered because you have nothing concrete to pin your grief to. In Western society there are no formalised rituals for acknowledging pregnancy loss and since the loss is in effect invisible to others they generally expect you to get over your sad feelings pretty quickly. To make the loss real and to honour the pregnancy, some couples choose to erect a memorial, plant a special plant or dedicate a day of the year to the memory of the baby they lost.

SANDS (Stillbirth and Neonatal Death Support) Australia is a support group of parents who have experienced the death of a baby through miscarriage or stillbirth or shortly after birth. These parents emphasise the importance of grieving after pregnancy loss and provide support and resources to couples who experience pregnancy loss. You can find SANDS on the net at www.sands.org.au.

A constant reminder of the loss

When you fall pregnant, your doctor gives you an estimated date of delivery — your due date. This date is supposed to be a happy occasion, something to look forward to — but not always. Maria experienced a pregnancy loss at 12 weeks gestation and described feeling profound grief at the time of her due date: She couldn't stop thinking that she should've been holding a baby in her arms but she wasn't. A friend commented on Maria's sadness and Maria explained that it was because of her due date. To Maria's consternation, her friend had trouble understanding her sadness: She expected Maria to have gotten over the pregnancy loss by that stage. Because of her friend's reaction, Maria stopped talking to her friends about how she was feeling, but for years afterwards the date reminded her of the baby she'd lost.

For some the mourning for a pregnancy loss is never really over, but for most people over time the acute pain is replaced by sadness that surfaces on particular occasions, like the anniversary of the due date. If you have trouble enjoying life again after a pregnancy loss, you may need help from a counsellor to move on.

Waiting and Hoping

IVF involves a lot of waiting for results and hoping that the treatment is going to work. Many outcomes from an IVF cycle — including whether you get pregnant or not — are out of your control and this can make you feel like your whole life is out of control.

Putting your life on hold

You may feel as though your life's on hold while you're on the IVF program and postpone big decisions like a job or career change, overseas travel, moving house or renovating while IVF rules your life. Even planning ahead for small things like a weekend away can be difficult — what if that's when your embryo transfer needs to happen?

Don't put everything on the backburner just because you're having IVF treatment. The outcome of IVF is always uncertain, so try to not let treatment rule your life. Get back in charge by making plans and sticking to them: Make IVF fit in with you rather than you fitting in with IVF.

Getting nowhere

Repeated IVF failure wears you down and makes you feel trapped. If the treatment doesn't work, all you can do to keep your hope of having a baby alive is to try again. Finding the mental energy to start all over again can be difficult, but you may feel that the alternative option — giving up on treatment — is even harder.

If you and your partner have the same drive to keep going with treatment you'll find things easier, but if one of you wants to quit and the other wants to keep going it's trickier. Unsurprisingly, research shows that the more similar partners in a couple are in their views about either continuing or discontinuing IVF, the easier they find it to make their decision. If you and your partner have different views about continuing IVF, try to see each other's point of view and endeavour to negotiate a way forward that you both feel works for you. For example, this may mean stopping after you've used up your frozen embryos or having one more shot at IVF.

Hope is an amazing driving force, but there may come a point in time when you run out of hope that the treatment is going to work. This can be very distressing because it means giving up on your dream to have children and being forced to make new life plans.

Sometimes you need help to face reality. Yes, you guessed it — an IVF counsellor can help you through the process of letting go and refocusing your life after IVF.

Deciding to stop treatment

Most couples find that being on the IVF program has some negative effects on their sex life, job, career and financial situation. In spite of this many couples keep trying, sometimes over a period of years. Others find the process of IVF too demanding and decide to not pursue treatment if they experience treatment failure.

The most common reason why couples stop treatment is that they're pregnant — a very good reason to stop! But for those who aren't so fortunate, the emotional demands of IVF are a much more common reason for discontinuing treatment than the physical burden of treatment. I talk more about the process of arriving at a decision to stop IVF treatment in Chapter 12.

Seeing Further Down the Track

Several studies have followed couples who had IVF for a period of time after their treatment. The good news is that within a few years of ending treatment, there are very few differences in terms of emotional wellbeing between those who had a baby as a result of treatment and those who didn't. Here are a few more results from these studies:

- **Infertility doesn't go away, even if you have a baby:** Interestingly, despite having a baby with IVF, many couples still think of themselves as infertile: It seems hard to shake off the experience of having fertility problems. That said, most couples who have an IVF baby know that they have to go through IVF again if they want more children, so it's understandable that they continue to think of themselves as infertile.

- **Life goes on, even if you don't have a baby:** The majority of couples whose IVF treatment doesn't work are able to move on and live satisfying lives. For many, in fact, it's a great relief when IVF is over because they can get on with the rest of their lives. They develop new life plans and goals, their spirits come back and life becomes pleasurable again. The sadness about being childless or having fewer children than planned may not go away completely, but after a while it no longer consumes so much time or mental energy.

- **Most couples who don't have a baby after IVF don't regret trying treatment:** Most couples who don't have a baby as a result of IVF feel that they've given it their best shot and are able to move on after finishing treatment. Many couples say that they tried IVF because they didn't want to later regret not having done everything they could to have a baby.

Chapter 12

Moving On When IVF Doesn't Work

Although the chances of having a baby with IVF have increased dramatically over recent years, the sad fact is that treatment still doesn't work for everyone. IVF clinics provide plenty of information about their 'success' rates, but you need to remember on the flip side that they also have a 'no success' rate.

Some couples fluke it first time around, but many couples need to try a few times before they strike it lucky and some couples never hit the jackpot. Clinics often talk about your 'cumulative chances', which may be something like your chances of having a baby after three stimulated cycles (see Chapter 5) and including any frozen embryos. But what happens if you're still not pregnant after several stimulated cycles? How long do you keep going with treatment? How do you know when there's no point continuing any more?

In this chapter, I discuss how you may arrive at a decision to stop treatment that feels right for you and how to move on with your life after treatment.

Taking Stock

If you receive a negative pregnancy test result or your cycle is cancelled because you don't have enough follicles or have no embryos to transfer, you have to decide whether you're going to try another treatment cycle. This decision may be difficult for you and your partner and you'll probably need input from your doctor and counsellors to help you through the decision-making process.

Reviewing your treatment

After you have an unsuccessful IVF cycle your doctor and the embryologist will put their heads together to try to figure out why the cycle failed and, more importantly, how they can change your treatment protocol to improve your chances of the treatment working next time. Your doctor then discusses the options with you and your partner. Your options may include tweaking the stimulation protocol to try to get more eggs, changing from day two to day five transfer, or using donor sperm, eggs or embryos instead of your own (see Chapter 13 for more about these options). Equipped with this information, you can then decide whether to give IVF another go.

However, after you've had several unsuccessful cycles, all the experts may be scratching their heads trying to think what else they can do to help you get pregnant. If you have trouble getting enough eggs, even on a high dose of follicle-stimulating hormone (see Chapter 6), or very few of your eggs fertilise normally (refer to Chapter 7), the experts may not have much to offer. Doctors are always keen to help their patients and when IVF doesn't work and you want to try again, your doctor will try hard to come up with something to improve your chances, but sometimes it's a bit like grasping at straws.

Whether or not your doctor has any more tricks up his or her sleeve to improve the outcome of your IVF treatment, you may reach a point when you've had enough. Only you will know when that happens.

 Finding medical solutions to your infertility problem is part of your IVF doctor's role, so your doctor may not broach the subject of stopping treatment with you. If you want to discuss this option, you may have to raise the issue with your doctor.

Getting off the merry-go-round

Deciding to stop IVF treatment can be difficult, because it may mean giving up on your dreams of becoming parents or having another child. That's why some couples just keep going with IVF, even if the chance of the treatment working is virtually zero. If this happens to you, you need someone to stop the merry-go-round so that you can both get off. Interestingly, in one study about IVF experience a whopping 79 per cent of women thought that couples should be counselled about the option to stop treatment.

If you're ready to stop treatment but your partner wants to keep trying, you may have to find a compromise, like having one last try. Try to work out something that you both feel okay with. Failing that, you may need help from a counsellor so you don't end up falling out with each other over the issue.

There's no right or wrong time to call it quits: The only important thing is to find the right time for *you*. Some couples make plans in advance about how many times to try IVF and stick to their plans; others need time to feel that they're ready to close the IVF door. Take the time you need, because this gives you a better chance to feel that you made the right decision.

Time to stop

Susan and Andrew joined their IVF program full of enthusiasm and optimism. However, unfortunately they weren't lucky and endured several unsuccessful treatment cycles. Not wanting to give up hope, they decided to try one last time. Amazingly, Susan's pregnancy test result came back positive, but their joy was short-lived when the scan two weeks later showed a smaller than expected foetus without a heartbeat. Naturally, they were both devastated. They also felt that they couldn't stop treatment because they'd finally seen some positive signs. However, another two unsuccessful cycles followed, so they decided to see the clinic counsellor. She helped them reach the conclusion that it was time they stopped treatment and got on with the rest of their lives. Looking back, Susan and Andrew know that they made the right decision and are grateful that the counsellor encouraged and supported them through the tough process of letting go.

Letting go

Deciding that you've had enough of IVF treatment can trigger all sorts of emotional responses. You may feel relieved about not having to go through a treatment cycle again, sad about not having the baby you want, angry with the clinic or lost about what to do next — or a mix of all these emotions. When you're actively having treatment this occupies a lot of your time and physical and emotional energy and you can keep thinking that next time it may work. But after you stop treatment you may find that it takes time to adjust to not being on the IVF program.

Dealing With Dashed Hopes

Part of the process of coming to terms with the fact that IVF hasn't worked for you is dealing with your disappointment and the disappointment of those close to you. IVF isn't just about hoping to have a baby — it's about hoping to experience parenthood and sharing this unique experience with your partner, hoping to extend the family tree and give your parents grandchildren, hoping to enjoy raising children together with your friends (who all already have children, of course) and looking forward to having your own grandchildren in the future.

Managing your disappointment

When IVF comes to nothing, you may have overwhelming feelings of disappointment. This is to be expected; after all, you've invested a lot of time, money, and physical and emotional capital without any return. It can take time to get over the disappointment and come to terms with not having a child or having fewer children than you want.

Over time, some of these negative feelings fade. In one study of women's IVF experience several years after treatment, only 12 per cent of the women who didn't have a baby agreed that their life had been negatively affected by IVF, while 91 per cent said that they were glad they'd tried IVF. But it can be difficult to totally give up hope of having a baby: 74 per cent of the women who didn't have a baby were still hoping to become pregnant and 68 per cent said that they would always be sad that they didn't have children.

Deep disappointment can sometimes feel like anger inside. If you're angry with your clinic, your doctor or your lack of success, for example, try talking to an IVF counsellor. Counsellors can help you deal with your anger so you can use this mental energy to get on with the rest of your life.

Handling your partner's disappointment

On top of coping with your own feelings of disappointment you may have to help your partner deal with his or her disappointment. When you're sad and hurting you may have difficulty extending support to your partner, but it's important that you work together to get through the disappointment stage as quickly as possible, so you can start to enjoy your life post-IVF.

Recognising your families' disappointment

Many of the people close to you will be disappointed that IVF hasn't worked for you. They've been keeping their fingers crossed hoping that your extraordinary effort would pay off and feel sad for you that it didn't. But they may also feel a bit sorry for themselves; for example, your mother may be disappointed that she won't become a grandparent or your sister may be sad that she won't be an aunt. If you already have children who were looking forward to having a sibling, they may feel that they've missed out on something they were looking forward to.

Although you can acknowledge others' disappointment, you have enough on your plate managing your own feelings and trying to help your partner and current children (if you have them), so try not to take on helping others as well. Your friends and family have to deal with their own feelings themselves and hopefully will soon realise that you need their love and support during this time, not their frustration.

Moving On

After you 'retire' from IVF you can get on with the rest of your life. So, what next? You may need time to adjust to the idea of not having children, but you may also find that the end of IVF is the beginning of new opportunities:

- **Establishing new life goals:** You now have to set new life goals that may or may not include children. Having had very little control over what happened to you while you were having IVF treatment, you may find it liberating to feel that you're back in charge and can make plans for the future. You can consider a career change or try to further the career you have, devote more time to a hobby or pursue new interests, travel the world or take on challenges such as working overseas. Whatever you choose to do, you're in the driver's seat.

✔ **Finding other ways to parent:** If having children in your life is still a top priority for you and your partner, you may want to look into alternative ways of parenting. For example, depending on your age you may consider adopting a child or acting as foster parents. Or you may prefer to develop closer relationships with your nieces and nephews or friends' children. You could also have children in your life by volunteering at the local hospital children's ward, helping out at the local school or church, or becoming a youth leader. It won't be the same as having your own children, but it can be very rewarding to be a mentor or confidante.

The adoption process varies between the states and is never easy. To find out more, talk to an IVF counsellor. The counsellor can also explain more about fostering children.

✔ **Living without children:** You may feel that if you can't have your own children, you want to make the most of being child-free rather than adopting or fostering children. If you decide to live without children, you're in good company: Increasingly, couples are choosing not to have children in order to be able to pursue other life goals.

Part IV
Pushing the Boundaries

Glenn Lumsden

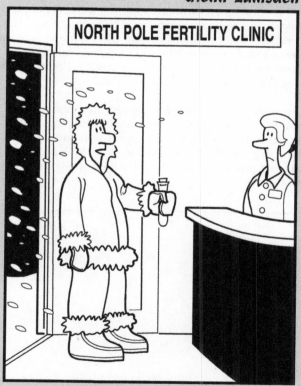

'Here's my sample. It's already frozen.'

In this part ...

*I*VF in its original form is straightforward: A couple's eggs and sperm are introduced to each other in the lab and the resulting embryos are placed in the woman's uterus a few days later. However, since its humble beginnings, IVF has evolved and today a lot of whizz-bang procedures are performed in IVF labs.

In this part, I explain third-party reproduction using a sperm donor or an egg donor, how freezing can widen your reproductive window of opportunity and how you can avoid passing on 'bad' genes. I also look at some promising research that may offer new opportunities in the future.

Chapter 13

Using a Donor

In This Chapter

▶ Adding a donor to your family tree

▶ Transferring the donor material

▶ Considering the legal side of donor conception

▶ Making sure donor conception is right for you

▶ Locating the right donor

▶ Working out how to tell your child

So-called third-party reproduction is an option you may want to consider if you can't use your own sperm or eggs (or both). The most recent data available from the Australian Institute of Health and Welfare show that about 650 babies are born annually in Australia and New Zealand as a result of donor gametes (sperm or eggs) or embryos. From a technical viewpoint, using donated gametes or embryos to help a couple to conceive is quite straightforward, but the psychological, social and legal aspects of gamete donation are much more complex.

In this chapter, I discuss why you may need a donor, the process for donor treatment and the legal side of donor conception. I also outline what you can expect from counselling, how you find a donor and how you decide who to tell about your donor conception, and when.

Finding Out That It May Take Three (or Four) to Tango

You may need donated gametes or embryos to conceive for any number of medical reasons. You'll probably try to have a baby with your own gametes first and then if that path is unsuccessful consider the option of using a donor. But you may know from the outset that the only way you can have a baby is by using donor gametes.

If you're a single or lesbian woman, you may want to use donor sperm for social reasons. In Chapter 4, I outline which Australian states allow the use of donor sperm for social reasons.

You can rest assured that potential donors are closely scrutinised by the clinic. At a minimum, the clinic asks that potential donors:

- ✔ Are aware of the potential risks of being a donor
- ✔ Are fit and healthy
- ✔ Are neither too old nor too young (precise ages vary between clinics)
- ✔ Are prepared to make information about themselves available to a child born as a result of the donation
- ✔ Provide a genetic and medical family history
- ✔ Undergo counselling
- ✔ Undergo screening for infectious and genetic conditions

Needing a sperm donor

You may need or prefer to use donor sperm for the following reasons:

- ✔ **Azoospermia:** Very few sperm are needed for the embryologist to be able to create embryos with the intracytoplasmic sperm injection (ICSI) procedure (see Chapter 7), but if you have azoospermia and so have no sperm at all, you need donor sperm.

- ✔ **Genetic condition:** If you know that you are a carrier of a severe genetic condition and don't want to risk passing this condition onto your child or children, you may prefer to use donor sperm.

- ✔ **HIV:** People infected with HIV can live very healthy lives thanks to the new drugs that are available, but men who carry the virus can theoretically pass on the infection to their partner and/or to their baby if their partner conceives with their sperm. So if you're HIV-positive, you may prefer to use donor sperm to protect your partner and baby.

  Some IVF clinics have developed specialised protocols for couples where the male partner is HIV-positive that allow his sperm to be used without risking passing on the infection to his partner or their baby. However, for the procedure to be safe the male partner has to have an undetectable or extremely low viral load.

- ✔ **Previously failed ICSI treatment:** If you have a low sperm count or a high proportion of abnormal sperm (see Chapter 1), you can usually conceive with the ICSI procedure, but if this procedure doesn't work you need donor sperm.

Needing an egg donor

You may need or prefer to use donor eggs for the following reasons:

- **Age-related infertility:** The older you are, the greater the probability that you won't respond to the hormone stimulation used in IVF treatment. In addition, the risk of chromosomal abnormalities in your eggs increases with your age, which means that even if you produce eggs in response to stimulation, the embryos may not be viable. So if you're over age 40 and have had disappointing results with IVF, you may consider using donor eggs.

- **Genetic condition:** If you know that you're a carrier of a severe genetic condition and don't want to risk passing this condition onto your child or children, you may prefer to use donor eggs.

- **Premature ovarian failure:** You're born with all the eggs that you'll ever have and at some point you'll run out of eggs (that's when menopause sets in). The average age for menopause is about 53, but sometimes women as young as their twenties run out of eggs, so-called *premature ovarian failure*. This condition is caused by a variety of factors, including a rare chromosomal anomaly called Turner's syndrome (where you have only one X chromosome instead of two), cancer treatment destroying your ovaries or your ovaries being surgically removed. If you have premature ovarian failure, you'll need donor eggs to conceive.

- **Recurrent miscarriage:** If you've suffered several miscarriages that are thought to be caused by an egg problem, donor eggs may help you to have a baby.

Opinion favours donor eggs

In a recent American study infertile women and men were asked about their attitudes towards donor eggs and donor sperm. Interestingly, both women and men were more sceptical towards using donor sperm than using donor eggs and believed that using donor sperm was more likely to have negative effects on their relationship and negative social consequences. They were more concerned about a lack of genetic link between the father and the child than between the mother and the child. Perhaps the fact that the mother carries the pregnancy and gives birth to the child is more important than her genetic link to the baby?

Needing an embryo donor

The best option if you need donor sperm *and* donor eggs is to use donor embryos. Although donor embryos are hard to come by, every year some couples decide to donate the frozen embryos that they no longer need to other couples (I talk about making this decision in Chapter 15). Such an amazing gift can help couples with complex infertility problems to have a family. Sometimes embryo donation is referred to as pre-conception adoption.

Transferring the Donor Material

Both donors and recipients need to think long and hard about the implications of donor procedures for themselves and their families before deciding to go ahead. But after all the parties involved have made up their minds, donor procedures are technically quite straightforward.

Donor sperm

Clinics store donated sperm in tiny straws in a tank of liquid nitrogen at a temperature of –196 degrees Centigrade. If the female partner doesn't have a fertility problem, the doctor uses a simple procedure called artificial insemination with donor sperm. At the time of your ovulation a small amount of donor sperm is thawed out and deposited at the top of your vagina or inside your uterus: If all goes to plan the sperm finds the egg, an embryo develops and nine months later you have a baby!

If a few attempts with artificial insemination don't do the trick or if the female partner also has a fertility problem, you can use donor sperm in an IVF cycle or an ICSI cycle (refer to Chapter 5 for more information on these procedures).

Because the risk of disease transmission is so high, clinics no longer use fresh sperm. Instead, sperm are frozen and the donor is retested for infectious diseases before the sperm are released for use.

Donor eggs

If you use donor eggs, the egg donor completes the first two parts of the IVF cycle and you complete the third, meaning that the donor undergoes hormone stimulation and egg collection (refer to Chapter 5 for more on these procedures). When the eggs have been recovered, your partner's sperm is added to the eggs and two to five days later, when the embryos are formed, you undergo embryo transfer. In preparation for embryo transfer you need to take a course of oestrogen tablets and progesterone, which ensures that the lining in your uterus is just right for the embryo to implant (for more on IVF drug protocols, refer to Chapter 6). After transfer you have to keep taking oestrogen and progesterone for up to ten weeks if you're pregnant, but after ten weeks your placenta produces enough hormones to maintain the pregnancy.

Donor embryos

Donated embryos are frozen, so all that's needed is for the timing of the embryo transfer to be perfect. This is calculated in exactly the same way as if you were using your own frozen embryos (refer to Chapter 5), depending on whether you have a regular menstrual cycle or an irregular menstrual cycle:

✔ **Regular cycle:** Just after ovulation is the best time to transfer the embryo, so you need to have an ultrasound examination and urine and/or blood tests to pinpoint the day of ovulation and then the embryo is transferred a few days later.

✔ **Irregular cycle:** If you don't ovulate every month, you have to get the lining in your uterus perfect for the embryo by either:

• Taking clomid tablets or having follicle-stimulating hormone injections to make you ovulate

• Taking oestrogen and progesterone to build up the lining

Understanding What the Law Says About Donor Conception

People contemplating donor procedures have to provide a lot of information about themselves so that in the future any child born as a result of a donation can find out about his or her origins. Federal law is silent on the issue of donor conception, and the amount and type of information required in relation to donor conception varies between the states and territories. Rules sometimes change, so if you're considering using donor gametes or embryos, you need to find out what the current situation is in the state where you plan to have treatment.

Some states keep central registers of donors and recipients, which enable children to find out information about their donor when they grow up and donors and recipients to access information about each other. In states that don't have central donor registers, the relevant clinic can help donors, recipients and donor-conceived children to find out information about each other.

✔ **Australian Capital Territory, Queensland and Tasmania:** The National Health and Medical Research Council's Ethical Guidelines on the Use of Assisted Reproductive Technology in Clinical Practice and Research guide clinics in these states regarding the information about donors, recipients and offspring that IVF clinics need to keep on record. The guidelines stipulate that clinics mustn't use gametes from donors who don't consent to identifying information about them being released because donor-conceived children have the right to know their genetic parents.

✔ **New South Wales, Victoria and Western Australia:** These states have central registers with information that IVF clinics are obliged to provide about the identity of donors, recipients and children born from donor procedures. The information can be accessed by a child once he or she turns 18.

✔ **Northern Territory and South Australia:** These states have no central registers but clinics have to keep records of donors, recipients and any offspring, and donor-conceived young adults are able to find out non-identifying information about their donor, such as hair and eye colour, blood group, height, education and interest. Identifying information is available to the donor-conceived young adult only if the donor agrees.

The amount of information that donors, parents and donor-conceived children can access depends on in which state or territory the donor procedure took place. In general, donors, parents and donor-conceived children can access *non-identifying information* about each other from the clinic where the treatment took place. For example, donors may be interested to know how many families have benefited from their donations and how many children have been born. Parents and donor-conceived children may want to know how old the donor is, whether other families have children from the same donor, what the donor's interests are, his or her hair and eye colour and so on.

Where information is available, donor-conceived children can access *identifying information* about the donor when they turn 18 years of age. From some registers the donor and the parents can also receive identifying information about each other, but only if the person to whom the information pertains gives consent.

Gametes and embryos must be donated for altruistic reasons only: Donors can't receive any payment or inducement for making a donation, although they can be reimbursed for any expenses they incur in relation to the donation, such as travelling expenses.

Thinking Carefully About Your Options

The most important issue in donor conception is that all those involved — donor(s) and recipients — think very long and hard about all the potential consequences of third-party reproduction for themselves, their family and any children who are born as a result of gamete or embryo donation.

Here's the bottom line if you're thinking of using donor gametes or embryos:

- **Eggs:** If you use donor eggs, your baby won't be genetically related to the female partner.
- **Sperm:** If you use donor sperm, your baby won't be genetically related to the male partner.
- **Embryos:** If you use donor embryos, the baby won't be genetically related to either of you.

Although many people aren't worried about this, some think that genetic links are very important. That's why clinics put a lot of effort into making sure that couples considering either receiving or donating gametes or embryos are given plenty of opportunity to consider the many issues that arise around donor conception before they go ahead. If you're thinking about using or donating gametes or embryos, expect in-depth discussions with an IVF counsellor to thrash out all the complexities involved in donor conception.

The donor doesn't have any legal obligations to a child born as a result of the donation; it's the couple who raise the child who are the child's legal parents.

Counselling is an essential part of the donor conception process. The idea is that you sit down with someone who knows all about donor conception and discuss issues such as:

- Future interactions between the donor and child
- How a donor will be found
- How the donation may impact on your relationship with the donor if he or she is known to you

✔ Practical and legal aspects of treatment

✔ The circumstances of the donation

✔ The impact of using donor gametes on your relationship with your partner

✔ The lack of a genetic tie to a child born after the procedure

✔ Who to tell about the donation — and when and how

✔ Your expectations of the procedure

Research shows that both donors and recipients find the counselling process more helpful than they think it will be, particularly with regard to gaining a better understanding of the legal side of donor conception, thinking about what to tell the child about being donor-conceived (and when) and whether the child is going to have contact with the donor in the future.

The whole point of counselling is to make sure that, as far as possible, everyone involved in donor conception is comfortable with the idea and aware of their responsibilities to a child who may be born as a result of the donation. The counsellor wants to be really certain that:

✔ A known donor isn't coerced or talked into being a donor.

✔ Both partners in the recipient couple feel that using a donor to have a baby is the right decision for them.

✔ Both partners in the recipient couple are aware of the importance of openness and are willing to consider the welfare of their child in relation to being informed about the way he or she was conceived.

✔ The donor informs his or her own children that they may have a biological half-sibling.

✔ The donor involves his or her partner in the decision to donate gametes.

✔ The donor is aware that he or she may be contacted by the child in the future.

If you decide to use donor eggs or sperm, the child created will be biologically related to *one* of you. The non-biological parent is the legal parent, but is this fact going to be a problem if you and your partner separate down the road? Is this issue something that one of you may fling in the other's face if the child has a serious health problem, or ends up in trouble with the law? Will the fact that one of you can see family features in your child's face while the other can't become a source of friction? You need to consider these questions, as well as any others that cross your mind, before you make the leap.

The counselling process sometimes makes donors and/or recipients aware of things they hadn't thought of or known about before. This can make them review their decision to be part of the donor process, which can be very upsetting for everyone involved. But it's far better for a participant to pull out before the event than to go ahead and regret their participation later down the track.

Finding a Donor

The clinic may recruit a donor unknown to you or you may recruit the donor yourselves. The greatest dilemma with donor conception is that there are never enough donors. This is unfortunate for all those who need donor gametes or embryos, but also understandable: Being a donor involves much more than just providing sperm, eggs or embryos, and most people aren't prepared to put themselves through the process of being a donor.

Using a donor selected by the clinic

Clinics with donor programs use advertising and public awareness campaigns to attract sperm, egg and embryo donors. Fortunately, some men step up to the plate and become sperm donors. Their sperm is frozen and can be used to help several couples over a long period of time. If you're using sperm donation, you'll be given non-identifying information about the potential donors to help you decide which donor to use. Most couples try to find a donor who has physical characteristics that are similar to those of the male partner.

Finding women prepared to donate eggs to someone they don't know is harder, but occasionally that happens and the clinic selects a recipient couple.

Embryo donors are couples who decide to donate frozen embryos that they aren't planning to use. In the hope that future contact between the recipient and donor families may be possible, clinics do their best to match the donor and recipient couples in terms of interests, race, religion and other characteristics.

Asking someone you know to be a donor

If you need an egg donor, your best bet is to BYO (bring your own). You may have a sister, cousin or friend who you feel comfortable approaching. If you're very lucky, someone close to you who knows you need donor eggs may offer to be a donor for you.

If you ask someone you know to be an egg donor for you, don't feel bad if she says no. Being an egg donor isn't for everyone and some women just can't bring themselves to do it — even if they'd love to be able to help you. The physical process of being an egg donor is much more complicated than for sperm donors. The egg donor has to go through several weeks of drug injections, blood tests and ultrasound scans, as well as the egg retrieval procedure.

Advertising for a donor

Many couples advertise to find an egg donor. This method relies on women reading the ad and deciding to respond, not because they expect payment or some other compensation, but because they want to help someone in need. If you're lucky enough to get a response and both of you and the donor feel right about going ahead after you've met, this way of finding an egg donor can work really well.

Some states have legislation in place regulating advertising for donors, so talk to your clinic counsellor before placing an ad. The counsellor can fill you in on any rules you need to follow and help you with the wording of your ad, to give you the best possible chance of finding a donor.

Deciding Whether to Tell

The *big* question in relation to donor conception is whether you tell your child about his or her donor origin. Some people feel strongly that children have the right to know their genetic origins, while others argue that it's best for children to grow up *not* knowing that they were conceived with the help of a donor. Counsellors and other professionals involved with donor procedures very much advocate for telling a child, because not telling can have devastating consequences, especially if the child finds out about being donor-conceived from someone other than the parents.

People with experience in this area believe that the right time for telling a child about his or her donor origin is sooner rather than later. Children told when they're young tend to accept the fact that they're donor-conceived as readily as they accept anything else they're told about their early life — it becomes part of their life story.

As if it wasn't hard enough to explain the facts of life to children, how do you explain something as complicated as third-party reproduction? You'll find the clinic counsellors full of wisdom about how to tell; they'll also point you to some excellent books that can help you find the right words when the time comes.

Secrets in families can be difficult to keep and secrets that emerge at the wrong time and in the wrong place can be very destructive. Don't feel ashamed about needing to use donor eggs, sperm or embryos to become parents. Most children would like to think that they were wanted that much!

Who to tell

In our research into donors and recipients who had counselling because they were contemplating donor procedures, my colleagues and I asked our study respondents who they thought should be told about using a donor. The recipients responded as follows:

✔ Child: 77 per cent

✔ Close family: 65 per cent

✔ Extended family: 27 per cent

✔ Close friends: 23 per cent

✔ Anyone: 9 per cent

Interestingly, the donors were more in favour of telling others than the recipients. For example, 91 per cent of donors thought that the child should be told about his or her donor origin.

Chapter 14

Using a Surrogate

Traditional surrogacy has been practised for centuries. Several Biblical accounts tell of women bearing children for others who couldn't have a family. Historically, the surrogate conceived via sexual intercourse with the child's father and the child was genetically hers as well as the father's. Today, however, gestational surrogacy involving IVF is the most common form of surrogacy. Embryos created in the lab with the infertile couple's eggs and sperm are transferred to the surrogate, who goes through the pregnancy and gives birth. After the baby is born the surrogate gives the baby to the infertile couple to raise as their own. In 2006 in Australia 20 babies were born as a result of surrogates carrying babies for infertile couples.

Although in the past surrogacy arrangements were informal agreements between those involved, today the infertile couple and the surrogate have to undergo intensive counselling, and sign a lot of legal paperwork. The infertile couple also has to be prepared for an enormous financial outlay and sometimes formal adoption procedures before they can raise the child as their own.

In this chapter, I discuss the process involved in surrogacy and outline how you can find out whether surrogacy is right for you. I also give you some tips on finding a surrogate.

Borrowing a Uterus

Most causes of infertility are treatable with IVF or ICSI, but in certain circumstances, that's not enough and you may need to find a woman who's willing to carry the pregnancy for you. These circumstances may include

- **Chronic illness:** If you're suffering from a chronic illness you may be advised that pregnancy can worsen your condition or that the drugs you take for your illness are harmful to a growing baby.

- **No uterus:** If you don't have a uterus, obviously you can't carry a pregnancy. You may have had a hysterectomy (surgery to remove the uterus) because of cancer or some other condition, or you may have been born without a functioning uterus.

- **Recurrent miscarriage:** If you can conceive but keep losing the pregnancies because of problems with your uterus, surrogacy may be an option.

- **Same-sex male couples:** If you're in a same-sex relationship, you may want to have a child that one of you is genetically linked to. In Victoria male gay couples who want to become parents (and don't want to adopt a child) can use the help of a surrogate. In other states, this isn't an option.

The infertile couple needing to use surrogacy to have a child are sometimes known as the *commissioning couple* and the surrogate is sometimes known as the *gestational carrier*. The genetic make-up of a child born after surrogacy varies depending on the surrogacy situation.

- **Using your eggs and sperm:** If your eggs and sperm are suitable, they can be used to form embryos in the lab with IVF (see Chapter 5) and these embryos are then transferred to the surrogate. This is known as *gestational surrogacy* and in this situation you are the child's genetic parents: The surrogate is genetically unrelated to the child.

- **Using donated eggs or sperm, or both:** If you don't have eggs but the surrogate is fertile and agrees to become pregnant with her own eggs, she can be inseminated with the commissioning father's sperm (if they're suitable) or with donor sperm. However, in this situation the surrogate is the genetic mother of the baby and this can make it harder for her to give up the baby after birth. As a result, the method used in Australia is for the surrogate to carry a baby that *isn't* genetically hers, using either an embryo formed with eggs from a donor other than the surrogate and sperm from the commissioning father (or a sperm donor), or an embryo donated by another couple.

What the Law Says About Surrogacy

For many years surrogacy was legal only in the Australian Capital Territory. In the last few years other states and territories have changed their laws and regulations to allow altruistic surrogacy and this is now legal in most parts of Australia. However, commercial surrogacy, where a woman is paid to carry a pregnancy, is banned throughout the country.

When a child is born a birth certificate is issued showing the names of the birth mother and her male partner, if she has one. In the case of surrogacy this causes a bit of a headache for legislators. However, in the Australian Capital Territory, Victoria and Western Australia parentage can be transferred to the commissioning couple, and by the end of 2010 this will also be the case in South Australia. While parentage orders are being developed in a number of states, this is a complex area with many parties involved, so it's important to obtain legal advice in relation to your particular situation.

In most states only heterosexual couples can use a surrogate, but in Victoria same-sex couples and single people (regardless of sex) are able to commission a surrogate.

Surrogacy in the media

The story of the first Australian baby born as a result of IVF and surrogacy made big headlines. Alice Kirkman was born in Melbourne in 1988. Her mother Maggie didn't have a uterus and her father Zev didn't have sperm, so Alice was conceived from one of her mother's eggs and donor sperm, and her aunt Linda carried the pregnancy and gave birth. After Alice's birth, surrogacy became illegal in Victoria, in spite of intense lobbying to allow altruistic surrogacy arrangements by Dr John Leeton, the doctor who made Alice's birth possible. So,

when Mr Stephen Conroy, a Labor Senator, and his wife Paula Benson who are from Victoria needed a surrogate, they had to go to New South Wales to go through the process. Ms Benson had suffered ovarian cancer and couldn't conceive or carry a pregnancy. One of her friends donated an egg, which was fertilised with Senator Conroy's sperm. Another friend carried the pregnancy and baby Isabella was born in 2006. Since then the Victorian law has changed and altruistic surrogacy is now legal.

Thinking Through the Surrogacy Option

Surrogacy is a big undertaking for all those involved and it goes without saying that the many potential medical, psychological, social and legal problems have to be carefully considered before you make the decision to go ahead and ask another woman to carry your baby.

You'll have several trips to the counsellor before a surrogacy agreement can proceed. Many parties are affected by a surrogacy agreement and the counsellor needs to ensure that they're all considered. This includes

- ✔ The child born as a result of surrogacy
- ✔ The commissioning couple
- ✔ The surrogate
- ✔ The surrogate's partner and children
- ✔ The extended families of the commission couple and the surrogate

The counsellor plays devil's advocate and paints all sorts of bad scenarios to allow you and the surrogate to imagine how you'd feel if any of the following happened and how you'd deal with it. For example, what would you do if:

- ✔ The surrogate doesn't get pregnant?
- ✔ The surrogate conceives twins?
- ✔ You and the surrogate disagree about prenatal testing?
- ✔ Prenatal testing shows an abnormality?
- ✔ The surrogate has health problems during the pregnancy?
- ✔ The baby has health problems or a disability?
- ✔ The surrogate has trouble giving up the baby?
- ✔ You disagree about the amount of contact between the surrogate and the child?

Finding a Surrogate

Your best hope for finding a surrogate is to ask a close friend or relative whether she's willing to help you. However, even if the woman you ask loves you and wants to help, carrying a baby for you may be something she feels she just can't do.

Asking someone you know

It takes a very special woman (with a special family) to agree to carry a pregnancy for another woman and most women would consider doing so only for a very close friend or relative. You may approach someone you know to see whether she's willing to help or you may be approached by a woman offering to help you. In either case, altruistic surrogacy presumes that a woman's decision to be a surrogate is motivated by her strong wish to help someone she cares for deeply and wants to have an ongoing close relationship with in the future.

One of the risks with surrogacy arrangements is that the surrogate goes through with the pregnancy and later regrets it. For example, if she carries a pregnancy and gives the baby to the commissioning couple to raise, then later discovers that she can't conceive or carry a pregnancy when she wants to have her own child, she may regret being a surrogate. To minimise the risks that the surrogate has any regrets later, the surrogate needs to be aged 25 or older (21 in New South Wales), have given birth before and preferably have completed her family.

Even if you have a written agreement with the surrogate, there's no way of enforcing that agreement should a dispute arise later over the child. Under the Australian legal framework it's difficult to legally recognise any woman as the mother of a child other than the woman who gives birth to the child, so if a dispute goes to court, the birth mother will usually be assumed to be the true and legal mother.

Heading overseas to find a surrogate

Couples who need a surrogate and aren't fortunate enough to know someone prepared to give them such a gift sometimes choose to go overseas and enter into commercial surrogacy agreements. In several parts of the United States and India, for example, agencies exist that broker commercial surrogacy agreements.

The Surrogacy Center Australia (www.surrogacyaustralia.com), an Australian surrogacy agency, offers to coordinate surrogacy arrangements from start to finish for couples and individuals who want to undergo the process of surrogacy in the United States or India.

Considering the costs

No Medicare rebate is available for surrogacy, so the financial costs of surrogacy for the commissioning couple are enormous and include the following costs:

- Consultations with health-care professionals to assess the suitability of the surrogate
- Counselling
- IVF treatment
- Legal fees
- Obstetric care
- Paediatric care

Furthermore, if you enter into a surrogacy agreement overseas, you also have to spend a vast amount of money on travel and fees for the surrogate mother and the agency that makes the arrangements.

Chapter 15

Putting Things on Ice

Gametes (sperm and eggs) and embryos can be frozen and stored for a very long time without being harmed, in a process known as *cryopreservation*. However, you pay for storage and there are rules for how long gametes and embryos can be stored (see the section 'Considering the Rules and Costs of Storage' later in this chapter).

A growing number of couples are completing their families as a result of IVF treatment but still have embryos in the freezer. That's why the number of embryos being stored in IVF clinics around Australia — and indeed, around the world — is increasing steadily. At some point couples with extra frozen embryos — known as *supernumerary embryos* — have to make the sometimes difficult decision about what to do with these embryos.

In this chapter, I explain why gametes and embryos are frozen and flag the rules and cost for storage. I also discuss your options regarding what to do with your supernumerary embryos.

Freezing Gametes and Embryos

Cryopreservation is really handy in many different situations, such as wanting to preserve some of your eggs or sperm before undergoing cancer treatment or when you have more than one or two really good-quality embryos after a stimulated IVF cycle. Although different methods are used for freezing gametes and embryos, after they're frozen they're stored in tanks of liquid nitrogen at a temperature of −196 degrees Centigrade. Material frozen at such a low temperature has no bioactivity, meaning that it can be frozen indefinitely without 'going off'.

Sperm

Men who are at risk of losing their fertility can freeze their sperm as an insurance policy for the option of having children in the future. You may want to freeze your sperm in the following instances:

- ✔ **As a back-up during IVF treatment:** When you undergo IVF treatment, you're asked to produce sperm 'on demand', which can be pretty nerve-racking. If you suffer from performance anxiety, you may be reassured by having some back-up frozen sperm, in case you can't produce the sperm sample when it's needed.

- ✔ **Before having a vasectomy:** Men who have a vasectomy clearly aren't planning to have more children. But because life circumstances change, sometimes in the most unexpected ways, and since vasectomy reversals aren't always successful, you may want to keep your options open by putting away some sperm before you have the 'snip'.

- ✔ **After undergoing testicular biopsy:** If you have very severe male factor infertility, sperm or small pieces of testicle can be removed surgically from your testicles and with the ICSI procedure your partner's eggs can be fertilised with your sperm (see Chapter 5). Any sperm or testicular tissue left over after ICSI can be frozen in case you need ICSI again.

- ✔ **Before starting cancer treatment:** Some types of cancer treatment, such as radiation and chemotherapy, can cause loss of fertility. So, if you need to undergo such treatment and think you may want to have children in the future, you can freeze some of your sperm before treatment.

The technique for freezing sperm has been around for a long time, and insemination with frozen and thawed donor sperm has been offered to couples with male factor infertility since the 1950s. Sperm freezing is simple in most cases: A special solution is added to the sperm to protect it from freeze damage and then small amounts of sperm are placed in vials, which are labelled and frozen, before being stored in tanks of liquid nitrogen.

Thawing sperm is a simple procedure, and sperm usually survive the freezing and thawing processes very well. Your doctor uses the thawed sperm either to inseminate your partner or for an IVF or ICSI procedure (see Chapter 5), depending on the cause of your fertility problem.

Eggs

You may consider freezing your eggs for several reasons:

- ✔ **Medical:** If you're diagnosed with cancer during your reproductive years you may be informed that the treatment will likely damage your ovaries and render you sterile. Such news is devastating for women who hope to become mothers one day. Depending on the type of cancer you have, egg freezing may be an option that provides you with a chance to have a baby in the future.

- ✔ **Moral:** You may oppose embryo freezing on religious grounds, in which case egg freezing can be an alternative.

- ✔ **Social:** As women age, the number and quality of their eggs decline. If you're young and don't yet have a partner or don't want to have children until you're older, you may opt to freeze your eggs in the hope that they can be used to help you have a baby when you're ready.

Although freezing sperm is a relatively simple process, freezing eggs is much more difficult. One of the problems with freezing eggs is that the egg is the largest cell in the body and therefore has a high water content, meaning that when an egg is frozen, damaging ice crystals form in the egg.

As a result, the success rate for freezing eggs is relatively low. The first freezing protocols offered about a 1 per cent chance of a live birth, although scientists have worked hard since then to improve freezing techniques. One US clinic now quotes a 50 per cent chance of having a baby if you're under 35 years of age and have 12 eggs frozen.

Egg freezing is sometimes advertised as 'fertility preservation', which sounds like you can just put your fertility on hold and use it later. This terminology is rather deceptive, because egg freezing offers only a limited chance of having a baby. If freezing your eggs is the only option you have of having a baby, it's certainly worth a go. However, if you want to have children and have a choice about when to have them, go for it while you're young: don't rely on using frozen eggs when you're older.

To freeze your eggs, you first have to go through hormone stimulation and the egg collection procedure (see Chapter 5). Obviously, the more eggs you produce, the greater your chances of at least one surviving the freezing and thawing processes and having all it takes to fertilise and develop into a healthy baby.

The fast freezing method (called vitrification) that has proven successful with embryos (see Chapter 7) has also proven useful for freezing eggs and ovarian tissue, and is increasingly being used by clinics that offer egg freezing.

When you're ready the embryologist thaws your eggs and inseminates those that survive (see Chapter 7). A few days later one or two healthy looking embryos are transferred — the rest is up to Mother Nature. If you have more embryos that look suitable for freezing (refer to Chapter 7 for what these embryos should look like), they can be frozen for later use.

Scientists are working to improve women's chances of conceiving using frozen eggs. One promising development involves freezing thin slices of ovarian tissue instead of mature eggs. When the woman is ready to have a baby, the ovarian tissue is transplanted back to her in the hope that it still has the capacity to grow follicles and develop eggs.

Embryos

Embryo freezing is an important part of every IVF program: About 30 per cent of all IVF births result from frozen embryos. The option to freeze embryos is mainly used by couples who have more than one or two healthy looking embryos after a stimulated cycle, but it's also used as an alternative to egg freezing. The chances of having a baby are much greater with frozen embryos than with frozen eggs, so women with a partner who're about to undergo cancer treatment are better off freezing embryos rather than eggs.

I describe embryo freezing techniques in Chapter 7, and in Chapter 8 I explain how your chances of having a baby can increase if you have frozen embryos.

The risks of freezing

The main risk with freezing is that the gametes or embryos become damaged in the freezing and thawing processes and so can't develop further. Generally, the not-so-perfect material runs the greatest risk of being damaged: The better the quality of the material when it's frozen, the better its chances of surviving unharmed as it's frozen and thawed.

Spending time in freezing conditions as an egg, sperm or an embryo doesn't seem to have any effect on babies born as a result of frozen gametes and embryos. Hundreds of thousands of babies have been born as a result of frozen sperm or embryos and they show no signs of being different from other babies. It's still early days for egg freezing, but so far there's no cause for concern about the health of babies born as a result of frozen eggs either.

Considering the Rules and Costs of Storage

To make sure that clinics aren't left with 'orphaned' frozen eggs, sperm or embryos, all Australian states and territories have laws and regulations regarding how long you can store frozen eggs, sperm and embryos.

- ✔ **New South Wales, Queensland, Tasmania and the Australian Capital Territory:** These states follow the National Health and Medical Research Council's (NHMRC) Ethical Guidelines on the Use of Assisted Reproductive Technology in Clinical Practice and Research, which stipulate that

  - When eggs and sperm are frozen, the maximum length of storage time should be stated in the consent form that the gamete provider signs before freezing. If the provider hasn't used the frozen material by the end of this time and hasn't consented to prolonging the storage time, the clinic should discard the gametes.

  - Embryos can be stored for a maximum of five years, but after that time consent can be renewed and storage extended for another five years.

- ✔ **South Australia and Northern Territory:** Although there's no legal storage time limit for eggs and sperm, clinics follow the NHMRC guidelines and state a maximum storage time in the consent form that the gamete provider signs. Embryos can be stored for a maximum of ten years and during this time clinics are required to contact couples every 12 months to ask them whether they want to continue keeping their embryos in storage.

- ✔ **Victoria:** The maximum storage time for eggs and sperm is ten years. Embryos can be stored for five years only, but couples can apply to the Victorian Assisted Reproductive Treatment Authority (www.varta.org.au) for an extension of this storage period.

- ✔ **Western Australia:** There's no storage time limit for eggs and sperm, but individual clinics have rules for how long they store gametes. Embryos can be frozen for a maximum of ten years, but the Reproductive Technology Council can extend this storage time under special circumstances.

Some couples decide what to do with their unused embryos before the maximum storage time is up, and some have trouble making a decision and wait until the storage time limit is up and they're forced to make a decision.

Unless you notify the clinic about your decision beforehand, the clinic contacts you a few months before the maximum storage time limit expires and asks you to decide what you want done with your embryos. If you're still unsure at this point, you may find talking over your options with the clinic counsellor helpful.

Remember to notify the clinic if you move house, so that the clinic can still contact you about your frozen embryos. Sometimes when clinics write to couples to let them know that their frozen embryos are approaching the storage time limit, they find that they are no longer at their last known address. 'Orphaned' embryos are destroyed after the maximum storage time limit expires.

All clinics charge a fee for keeping your frozen gametes or embryos — usually a few hundred dollars per year. The cost of storage is not refundable by Medicare or private health insurance schemes. Although this amount may seem quite small in the scheme of things, usually it's enough to prompt couples to make a decision about their embryos if they're not planning to use them.

Deciding What to Do With Your Surplus Embryos

Tens of thousands of embryos are stored in freezers in IVF labs around Australia. Initially you freeze your embryos to improve your chances of having a baby. After several years, however, you may have all the babies you want and don't need the rest of your frozen embryos. Occasionally there are sadder reasons why couples don't use their frozen embryos; for example, separation or chronic illness may prevent you from having your embryos transferred. Irrespective of why you don't use all your frozen embryos, at some point you need to make a decision about what to do with those that are left in storage.

Knowing your options

Before you agree to freeze any embryos your IVF doctor asks you to think about what you'll do if you end up with more embryos than you need and explains your options. The vast majority of couples use all their frozen embryos, so for them such a question is hypothetical. However, if you have to make a decision about the fate of your embryos, this can be difficult.

Some people see an embryo as just a cluster of cells that they don't attach much significance to, whereas others see an embryo as a potential human being. Your view about what an embryo represents is likely to influence your decision about what to do with your left-over embryos and how easy or difficult you find making the decision.

You have three choices:

- ✔ **Discarding:** If you decide to discard your embryos, the embryologist removes the straw containing the embryos from the freezer and discards it as medical waste. You may prefer to take the straw home so that you can dispose of it in a way that feels right for you.

- ✔ **Donating to research:** Embryologists are always trying to find ways to improve IVF results and by donating your frozen embryos to research you can help the embryologists to perfect their culture techniques or to find out more about embryo development.

- ✔ **Donating to another couple:** For couples with complex fertility problems who need both donor sperm and donor eggs, the perfect solution is to receive an embryo from someone who decides to donate their embryos.

Tackling the dilemma

With some colleagues, I carried out a study of 123 couples who had frozen embryos that they didn't intend to use. We asked the couples what they planned to do with their embryos and how easy they found making their decision.

- ✔ Half of the couples said that they knew what they wanted to do with their embryos. The partners in each couple either didn't find making the decision difficult or were able to come to a joint decision that they both were happy with.

- ✔ The other half said that they really tussled about what to do with their embryos and found making the decision quite difficult and distressing.

Discarding the embryos

About 30 per cent of the couples decided to discard their embryos. The most common reason given for this decision was that they didn't want to donate their embryos to another couple, because any baby born as a result would be a full sibling to their own children. The second most common reason was that the couples didn't want any research to be performed on their embryos.

Donating the embryos to research

More than 40 per cent of the couples decided to donate their embryos to research in order to improve IVF outcomes. The most common reason for this decision was a desire to help advance science and a second reason was that the couples didn't want to waste their embryos by discarding them.

Some years ago scientists were able to grow colonies of embryonic stem cells from frozen embryos. Embryonic stem cells have the potential to become any kind of tissue in the body and scientists hope that one day stem cells will help them to find cures for chronic diseases such as diabetes and Parkinson's. Stem cell research is a very emotive issue: In general, people either don't like the idea of embryos being used in this way or they're all for it. Among the couples in our study, 69 per cent approved of embryo donation for stem cell research.

Donating the embryos to another couple

Donating frozen embryos to another infertile couple was the least common decision among the couples we surveyed — only 16 per cent were willing to do this. The couples that made this decision all said that their reason was to help another couple, but many also said that they wanted to give their embryos a chance at life.

The list of couples waiting for donor embryos is huge, but unfortunately very few embryos are available for donation. In 2006, 176 couples received donor embryos and 29 of them were lucky enough to have a baby as a result. Research shows that if couples have a say in who receives their embryos, they're more willing to go ahead and donate their embryos to another couple. For example, the donating couple may have a preference for the recipient couple to follow a certain religion or to be from a particular ethnic background.

Disagreeing about what to do with the embryos

The most difficult situation that can arise is when both partners in a couple disagree about what to do with their frozen embryos. In our study, 56 per cent of couples said they were in complete agreement about what to do, 37 per cent were able to come to a joint decision after some discussion, but 7 per cent simply couldn't agree and didn't know how to resolve their disagreement. In most cases such disagreement resulted from only one partner in a couple wanting more children. Under these circumstances, arriving at a decision that both partners feel happy with is extremely difficult, but sometimes talking to a counsellor or taking more time to think about what to do can help you to reach agreement.

Chapter 16

Avoiding Passing on 'Bad' Genes

In This Chapter

▶ Finding out what's in your genetic baggage

▶ Checking the genetic health of your embryos

Some health problems have a genetic origin, which means that they can be passed on from one generation to the next. Genes are the building blocks of life and heredity, and scientists worked for decades to identify the many thousands of genes in the human body. Finally, in 2003 the Human Genome Project was completed, so now scientists know which genes are responsible for certain medical conditions and where on the chromosomes these genes are located.

In this chapter, I briefly overview how IVF techniques can help you avoid passing on serious chromosomal and genetic conditions to your children.

Understanding the Genetic Lottery

Every cell in the human body has 46 chromosomes, made up of 23 pairs. You inherit one chromosome in each pair from your mother and the other chromosome from your father. Of the 23 pairs of chromosomes, there are 22 pairs of autosomes (chromosome pairs 1–22) and one pair of sex chromosomes, XX for women and XY for men. Chromosomes are made up of thousands of genes. Sex chromosomes carry the genes that transmit sex-linked traits and conditions; autosomes carry the genes that transmit traits and conditions other than those that are sex-linked. Your genes determine the colour of your eyes and hair and the shape of your toes, but also to a large extent your health.

In the process of reproduction, things sometimes go wrong and an embryo may end up with one chromosome too many or one chromosome too few. Usually such an error isn't compatible with life and the embryo dies.

However, sometimes the embryo survives and a baby is born. For example, babies born with Down syndrome have an extra chromosome 21, and they commonly have a range of health problems throughout their lives, including intellectual disability.

If you know that a certain genetic condition runs in your family or you know that you or your partner is affected by a genetic condition, you can see a geneticist or a genetic counsellor before you try to have a baby, to find out about the risk of passing on the condition to your offspring.

However, sometimes you may unknowingly be a carrier of a defective gene and you don't find out that you have a problem until it's too late — when your child is born with a genetic condition. If you plan to have more children, you can consult a geneticist or a genetic counsellor to discuss the risk of having another child affected by the same condition.

Undertaking Pre-implantation Genetic Diagnosis

You can undergo several tests when you're pregnant to make sure that the foetus has the right number of chromosomes and, if you're at risk of passing on a severe genetic condition, that the foetus is unaffected by this condition. However, although this is all well and good if the test results come back normal, if the results reveal a problem with the foetus, you then have to make the heart-wrenching decision whether to terminate the pregnancy or continue knowing that your baby has a potentially severe health problem.

To avoid this dilemma, you can opt for your embryos to be tested in the lab *before* you fall pregnant. To do this, you undergo an IVF treatment cycle (I explain the cycle in Chapter 5) and then have the resultant embryos tested, to make sure that only those that aren't affected by the condition tested for and have the right number of chromosomes are transferred. This is called *pre-implantation genetic diagnosis* — or PGD for short.

Some people oppose testing of embryos and argue that it can lead to 'designer babies', whereby embryos are selected based on whether they have certain *desirable* genes such as an athletic gene or an academic gene. However, athletic or academic talent doesn't come from a single gene and not only that — such talent very much depends on the environment in which the child grows up. So PGD can't actually be used to make 'designer babies'.

Testing for severe genetic conditions

Some genetic conditions cause extreme and lifelong suffering. These include

- ✔ **Beta-thalassaemia:** This blood disorder leads to a lack of oxygen in many parts of the body and anaemia, which can cause weakness, fatigue and more serious complications.

- ✔ **Cystic fibrosis:** This life-threatening genetic disorder predominantly affects the lungs and digestive system. People with cystic fibrosis produce an abnormal amount of thick mucus that blocks the airways, leading to repeated lung infections.

- ✔ **Fragile X:** This genetic disorder results in a range of physical, intellectual, emotional and behavioural problems.

- ✔ **Huntington's disease:** This genetic disorder affects muscle coordination and some cognitive functions.

- ✔ **Spinal muscular atrophy:** This genetic disorder results in progressive muscle wasting and weakness.

Scientists have discovered exactly where the faulty genes that are responsible for these severe conditions are located, so now highly specialised embryologists can use PGD to test embryos to find out whether they're affected by these disorders or not.

Some genetic conditions, such as haemophilia and Duchenne muscular dystrophy, affect only boys, not girls. If you have a known risk for one of these so called X-linked diseases, embryologists can determine the sex of your embryos and transfer only 'girl' embryos. However, sex selection for so-called family balancing reasons — where a female (or male) embryo is chosen because the parents specifically want a girl (or boy) — can't be carried out in Australia: In 2005 the Australian Health Ethics Committee ruled that embryo sex selection is permissible for medical reasons only.

Using PGD for other reasons

If you have numerous good-quality embryos transferred without success or you miscarry several times, your embryos may be *aneuploid*, meaning that they have the wrong number of chromosomes. If your doctor thinks that this may be the case and your clinic performs PGD, you may be offered the procedure to see whether you have a high number of aneuploid embryos and to ensure that aneuploid embryos aren't transferred.

If you've experienced several miscarriages, your doctor may suggest that you and your partner have a blood test to determine whether the miscarriages were the result of a balanced translocation (where a piece of chromosome breaks off and attaches to another chromosome). People with a balanced translocation don't normally have health problems as a result of the translocation because they have the full complement of genetic material — but their sperm or eggs may have some missing or extra genetic material, which can lead to miscarriage. If your miscarriages were the result of a balanced translocation, your doctor may suggest that you opt for PGD of your embryos to check that the embryos have the correct amount of genetic material before being transferred.

Performing PGD

PGD is performed at the bigger IVF clinics only, because the procedure requires extremely sophisticated lab equipment and specially trained and very skilled embryologists. If you have a known or suspected genetic condition and your doctor thinks PGD can be used to avoid passing this condition to your baby, you and your partner follow these steps:

1. **Undergo a genetic test:** To check whether one or both of you carry the 'faulty' gene or have a balanced translocation, you have a blood test or buccal swab (whereby cells are collected by swabbing the inside of your cheek).

2. **Have a consultation with a geneticist or genetic counsellor:** At this meeting the geneticist discusses the results of your genetic tests and advises whether PDG is feasible in your situation.

3. **Meet with your IVF doctor:** Your doctor explains what PGD involves and outlines the pros and cons of the procedure.

If you decide to go ahead with PDG, you undergo an IVF treatment cycle up to and including embryo development in the lab (refer to Chapter 5), so that ideally several embryos are available for testing. The PGD process then proceeds as follows:

1. **The embryologist performs embryo biopsy:** Three days after egg retrieval, when the developing embryos have about eight cells each, the embryologist removes one or two cells from all the embryos that have developed for testing.

   Note: Some clinics wait until five days after egg retrieval so that they can remove several cells from each embryo.

2. The embryologist carries out genetic testing on the chosen cells:

- If your embryos are being tested for a genetic condition, the embryologist determines whether the faulty gene is present or not in each cell.

- If your embryos are being tested for the right number of chromosomes, the embryologist verifies that the cells have the correct number (two) of the eight chromosomes that can be tested.

If PGD reveals healthy embryos, on day five after egg retrieval you have one or two embryos transferred. Additional healthy embryos can be frozen (see Chapter 5 for more information on freezing your embryos). After a couple of weeks of crossing all your fingers and toes, you have a pregnancy test, which hopefully comes back positive!

Understanding the limitations of PGD

The fact that some cells are removed from the early embryo in the PGD procedure doesn't appear to have any negative effects on either the embryo's chance to implant and develop or the health of the resultant baby. However, you need to be aware of the following before you agree to PGD:

- ✔ If you're having PGD to check which of your embryos has the right number of chromosomes but have only one or two embryos available, your doctor may advise you *not* to go ahead with the procedure. This is because it's more beneficial to transfer these embryos without subjecting them to biopsy.

- ✔ If you're having PGD because you risk passing on a genetic condition and want to be sure that the baby is unaffected, PGD may be done even with a small number of embryos.

- ✔ Only good-quality embryos can be tested, so if on day three your embryos haven't developed to the eight-cell stage or have a lot of fragments (refer to Chapter 7 where I explain more about good-quality embryos and what constitutes poor quality), PGD can't be carried out.

- ✔ Test results can be incorrect or inconclusive. For example, embryos can have a mixture of normal and abnormal cells, so even if the few cells that are tested are okay, the rest of the embryo may not be. And occasionally, PGD results aren't as clear as desired and can be difficult to interpret.

- ✔ The fact that PGD shows that an embryo is free of a certain disease doesn't guarantee that the embryo is free of other genetic conditions.

✔ Very rarely, an embryo is damaged during the embryo biopsy procedure and stops growing, so it cannot be used.

✔ To verify the PGD result, clinics recommend that you have prenatal diagnosis if you become pregnant after PGD. This is because the accuracy of prenatal testing results is higher the more cells that are tested. With PGD, only one or two cells are tested, whereas with chorionic villus sampling and amniocentesis thousands of foetal cells are tested and these procedures have 99 per cent accuracy.

Your doctor advises you not to have unprotected sex during the cycle in which your embryos undergo PGD, in order to eliminate the risk that you conceive spontaneously and have a foetus with a genetic or chromosomal defect.

Chapter 17

Looking at Future Possibilities

From humble beginnings, assisted reproductive technologies have come a long way. The birth of the first IVF baby, Louise Brown, in the United Kingdom in 1978 was the culmination of many years of research. In those days no fertility drugs were used — doctors simply waited round the clock for the right time to retrieve the one and only egg that a woman releases every month, even if this meant performing surgery (that's how eggs were retrieved then) in the middle of the night. And, if doctors did manage to catch a woman's elusive egg, getting it to fertilise and divide was another major hurdle because lab culture systems were less than perfect. So, in the early days of IVF women went through an awful lot for only a microscopic chance of having a baby.

Since then, research has resulted in great improvements in every aspect of IVF: Fertility drugs ensure that women have plenty of eggs; doctors use ultrasound to retrieve eggs safely; improved cultures allow healthy embryos to form and grow; and better transfer techniques help doctors to deliver embryos undamaged into the uterus. But the work to improve IVF outcomes is never over and scientists continue to look for new ways to improve success rates and find new treatment options for those who can't be helped with current techniques.

In this chapter, I describe some recent developments and emerging areas of research that hopefully will help deliver improved IVF outcomes in the future.

Getting Eggs Without Stimulating the Ovaries

Hormone stimulation is one of the cornerstones of modern IVF, but for women with polycystic ovaries or polycystic ovarian syndrome who have many tiny follicles in their ovaries, the stimulation protocol can be difficult to manage and they risk over-responding to the drugs and developing ovarian hyperstimulation syndrome (OHSS) (see Chapter 10). Embryologists are currently perfecting a technique known as in-vitro maturation (IVM) to allow such women to have IVF without hormone stimulation. Using IVM, the doctor retrieves immature eggs from tiny follicles in the woman's ovaries and then the embryologist places these eggs in a special culture medium for a few days to allow them to mature before introducing them to the partner's sperm. So, no need for injections and no risk of OHSS — sounds perfect.

At this stage, only a few clinics have the know-how to perform IVM and work still needs to be done to increase the procedure's success rate. But as the technique is refined and results improve, the use of IVM for certain groups of patients is likely to become more widespread in the coming years. About 1,000 babies have been born from IVM to date and all the signs point to them being as healthy as other children.

Although some predict that IVM will become the IVF treatment of choice in the future, for women who don't have a large number of tiny follicles in their ovaries, hormone stimulation is likely to continue to be their best bet to get several eggs for IVF.

Identifying the Most Viable Embryos

The majority of embryos created in IVF labs — and indeed many of the embryos that come into being as a result of good old-fashioned sex — don't survive to develop into babies. Embryologists grade embryos based on their appearance (see Chapter 7) and good-looking embryos have a greater chance of developing into babies than not so good-looking embryos. But there's more to it than looks alone because even the best looking embryos don't always result in pregnancies and sometimes embryos that don't look so flash continue to develop into healthy babies.

Wouldn't it be great to know which of your embryos has the greatest potential to develop into a baby so that you don't have to waste precious time transferring non-viable embryos? That's exactly what embryologists are currently trying to do. Growing embryos produce substances that embryologists can measure in the culture medium where the embryos grow, and embryologists are getting better and better at using this information to help them select the most viable embryos for transfer. In the future, embryologists hope to be able to select only the most viable embryos for transfer and/or freezing.

Making the Embryos Stick

Some couples undergo embryo transfer after embryo transfer without getting pregnant. This implantation failure means that, for some couples, IVF just doesn't seem to work. Implantation failure is a devastating event for these couples and is therefore the focus of much research. Scientists are exploring several possible reasons for implantation failure, including

- Microscopic blood clots may disrupt the process of implantation
- The mother's immune response may prevent the embryo from implanting
- The uterine lining may not have the right hormone profile for implantation
- Toxins from a past or current subclinical infection in the uterus may prevent implantation

Scientists are hoping to pinpoint the exact causes of implantation failure and then find ways to remedy these issues in order to improve the chances of embryos implanting successfully.

In addition, scientists have identified certain gene patterns among women who experience implantation failure and are working on isolating these patterns as a predictor of IVF success. So, in the future, it may be possible to look at your gene pattern before you start IVF treatment in order to get a good estimate of your chances of having a baby with IVF. If your odds are really bad, you may decide not to go ahead with the treatment.

Freezing Young Eggs and Having Babies Later

To some women, the idea of freezing their eggs while they're in their twenties when the eggs are at their best and then using the frozen eggs when they find Mr Right is very attractive. Up until recently this option wasn't viable, because very few eggs survived the freezing and thawing processes. However, in the last few years scientists have made much progress and egg freezing is looking more and more promising (refer to Chapter 15 for more about the freezing process).

So, in the future theoretically women could freeze their eggs when they're in their twenties and relax knowing that if they don't find Mr Right until they're in their late thirties or early forties, all is not lost on the baby front. However, it's unlikely that using egg freezing to delay childbearing will become widespread because it's a pretty costly and complicated way of doing something that nature designed to be easy and enjoyable!

Offering Low-cost IVF in Developing Countries

IVF and other assisted reproductive technologies are very high-tech and expensive forms of treatment that are available almost exclusively in developed countries. However, the personal tragedy of childlessness is no different for men and women in developing countries. In fact, in some cultures women who can't have children may risk public humiliation, divorce, abandonment or withdrawal of food and financial support — even if their infertility is due to a sperm problem.

As a result, the Low Cost IVF Foundation has developed a very simplified IVF protocol that's being trialled in some African countries. The idea is that one IVF cycle shouldn't cost more than $300. To keep costs down, the protocol:

- ✔ Relies on cheaper drugs — rather than using expensive drugs to stimulate egg production, women in the trial take a five-day course of clomiphene citrate tablets (refer to Chapter 6), which usually results in two to four eggs being available at egg collection

- ✔ Restricts monitoring to one ultrasound examination

- ✔ Uses very basic embryo culture systems

- ✔ Transfers just one embryo to avoid multiple pregnancies

If this protocol produces reasonable rates of success, in the future IVF could become a feasible option for infertile couples in poorer countries.

You can follow the progress of this initiative on the Low Cost IVF Foundation's website (www.lowcost-ivf.org).

Curing Chronic Diseases

Many years of IVF-related research led to the discovery of embryonic stem cells about a decade ago. Embryonic stem cells, which are produced by embryos, have the potential to develop into any type of cell in the body — for example liver, brain or skin — and scientists all over the world are working very hard to find ways of using these cells to repair and regenerate tissue that's affected by chronic disease. Many believe that in time diseases like diabetes, Parkinson's and Alzheimer's will be cured using stem cell technology. Apart from relieving human suffering, if stem cell therapy proves successful the health-care cost savings would be enormous. However, the issue is extremely controversial and debates about the ethics of using embryonic stem cells are ongoing worldwide.

Couples at risk of passing on serious genetic conditions to their offspring can take advantage of pre-implantation genetic diagnosis or PGD (refer to Chapter 16) to ensure that only healthy embryos are transferred. If PGD identifies any of a couple's embryos as having a genetic disease, the couple may decide to donate the embryos for research, giving scientists an opportunity to study these diseases. By comparing embryonic stem cells extracted from embryos affected by a genetic condition with embryonic stem cells from healthy embryos, scientists hope to gain insight into how various genetic conditions develop and how they can be treated.

Part V
Beyond IVF

Glenn Lumsden

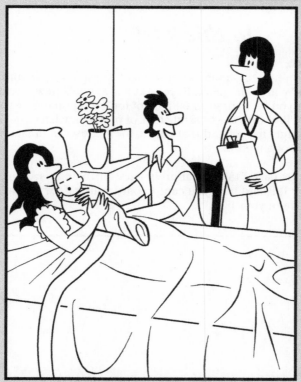

*'With a bit of scientific help,
the miracle of life just got even
more miraculous.'*

In this part ...

Congratulations: IVF treatment worked for you and you're pregnant! Beyond IVF is a whole new world, one you've wanted to be part of for a long time. But you may find that the blissful state of pregnancy isn't so blissful after all and that caring for a baby can in fact be a bit of a nightmare.

In this part, I talk about pregnancy, birth and parenting after IVF, and how you can prepare yourself for this new phase of your life.

Chapter 18

Jumping For Joy: Baby On the Way!

After all the trials and tribulations of infertility and IVF treatment you've finally reached your goal: You're pregnant! The end of your infertility journey marks the beginning of a new and exciting phase in your life. The transition to parenthood begins with pregnancy, and you have a lot of work to do to get ready for the birth and your new life as a parent.

Research shows that there are many similarities, but also important differences, between women who conceive with the help of IVF and those who conceive the 'old-fashioned' way in how they experience pregnancy, childbirth and mothering. In this chapter, I outline what's special about being pregnant after IVF and give you a few tips about what you can do to prepare for parenthood.

Finding Your Pregnancy Hard to Believe

When you conceive with the help of IVF you find out about your pregnancy much sooner than do couples who conceive spontaneously. So at first you may find it hard to believe that you're finally pregnant, especially if you don't have any pregnancy symptoms. However, after you've actually seen the little foetus on your six-week ultrasound examination, your pregnancy starts to feel more real. That's when you may find that your worrying about the outcome of every step in the IVF process becomes worrying about the outcome of your pregnancy!

Wondering whether your baby will be okay

From time to time every woman thinks about the wellbeing of her unborn baby and hopes that her baby will be born healthy. After IVF treatment, you may be even more preoccupied thinking about whether your baby is developing normally and will be okay. For some women who conceive with IVF, worry about the welfare of their baby stops them from fully enjoying the fact that they're pregnant — especially in the first few weeks of their pregnancy. However, these feelings don't usually last and in the second half of pregnancy, when they feel the baby moving, most women worry less and often feel quite blissful.

Some parents-to-be don't dare feel joyful about their pregnancy in case it's taken away from them. The fact that a small proportion of pregnancies don't have a happy outcome shouldn't stop you from feeling delighted about being pregnant and full of anticipation about becoming a parent: You've earned it! Allowing yourself to enjoy your pregnant state won't increase your risk of losing the pregnancy.

Telling others

So, when is the right time to tell the world (or those close to you, at least) that you're pregnant? It depends on what feels right for you. Some couples tell everyone as soon as they get the result of the pregnancy test, while others prefer to wait until their pregnancy is well under way. If you don't have any bleeding and see a foetus with a heartbeat in your uterus at your six-week scan, you can feel pretty confident that things are going according to plan, and so this may be a good time to share your exciting news.

Cutting the Ties With Your IVF Team

When you undergo IVF treatment you're in constant contact with the members of your IVF team. But after your six-week scan confirms your pregnancy, you have to say goodbye to your team and move onto the obstetric team for antenatal care. However, the obstetric team members usually don't want to see you until several weeks after your first scan and during this wait some couples describe feeling a bit abandoned, unsure who to turn to with questions they have.

If you're worried about something before you have your first antenatal visit, contact your IVF nurse: The IVF nurses are always willing to help, and if they can't answer your queries, they'll point you in the direction of someone who can.

Who looks after you now?

To make sure that everything is going well with you and your baby during your pregnancy, you have regular antenatal care check-ups. Your antenatal care alternatives depend on your preference, whether you have private health insurance, whether you have a straightforward or complicated pregnancy, and where you live. The options are

- ✔ **GP shared care:** Your antenatal care is shared between your GP and midwives and obstetricians in a public hospital.

- ✔ **Independent midwife:** In some places you can find an independent midwife to look after you. Independent midwives are practitioners in their own right and specialise in normal pregnancy care.

- ✔ **Midwifery care in a public hospital:** You see a midwife in a public hospital for most of your antenatal clinic visits, but for some visits you're also examined by an obstetrician.

- ✔ **Private obstetrician:** If you have private health insurance, you can see the obstetrician of your choice. Your obstetrician cares for you from early in your pregnancy until after your baby is born.

- ✔ **Public hospital antenatal clinic:** In some hospitals, clinics staffed with obstetricians and midwives with expertise in detecting and managing different types of pregnancy complications are available for women with high-risk pregnancies.

Wanting less and wanting more

A few years ago some colleagues and I carried out a large study of almost 200 women's experiences of pregnancy, childbirth and mothering post-IVF. We followed the women from early in their pregnancies until their children were 18 months old. These women very kindly shared their experiences by completing questionnaires in early and late pregnancy, and three, eight and eighteen months after childbirth.

Two very different sentiments about antenatal care were expressed in our study:

✔ Nina, who was 34 and fell pregnant with her first baby after two IVF cycles, said: 'All I want is to feel "normal" again. The whole deal with getting pregnant with IVF makes it all feel so technical, so now that I'm pregnant I want to see as few medical people as possible and just enjoy the natural process of pregnancy.'

✔ Sylvia, who was 39 and had experienced two miscarriages before finally having an ongoing pregnancy on her fifth IVF cycle, stated: 'I feel so reassured every time I see my doctor, and best of all is to have a scan where I can see for myself that the baby is alive and growing. After my visits I feel relaxed and happy knowing that all is going well but after a week or so I start to worry about the baby again and count the days until I have my next antenatal visit.'

You're like everyone else now but . . .

When you're pregnant you're theoretically like every other pregnant woman: Suddenly, you're part of mainstream society again after all the attention and medical interventions you've had during your IVF treatment — and this can take a bit of getting used to. On the one hand, you may feel a bit worried about not having constant medical check-ups; but on the other hand, you may feel relief about being like everyone else again.

Getting Prodded and Probed

Antenatal care is all about monitoring the health of mother and baby so that any problems with the pregnancy are detected early and managed effectively. Women who conceive with the help of IVF often have more antenatal visits than women who conceive spontaneously. Partly this is because IVF mums are older and therefore are more likely to have pregnancy complications (see Chapter 10), to carry twins and to be first-time mums.

But I think a few extra visits are often scheduled in for 'peace of mind' — the doctor's and yours!

Making decisions about antenatal screening and testing

Early on in your pregnancy you have a lot of routine blood tests to determine your blood group and haemoglobin levels and to test for certain infections. You're also offered two screening tests — a blood test and an ultrasound examination — to check for chromosomal abnormalities in the foetus such as Down syndrome (for more on different types of chromosomal abnormalities, refer to Chapter 16). You don't have to take these tests, and some couples choose not to. If you're unsure about taking the tests because you're worried about the results, talk to your doctor.

Screening tests give you an estimate of the risk of your baby having a chromosomal abnormality but the results aren't definitive. If both tests are normal, the risk is minimal, but if at least one test isn't normal, you'll be offered diagnostic testing — either chorionic villus sampling (CVS) or amniocentesis — whereby cells from the foetus are tested. Whereas screening tests give you a 'probably' result, diagnostic testing gives you a definite 'yes' or 'no' result.

Screening tests aren't always conclusive and your doctor may recommend that you undergo diagnostic testing based on your screening test results. The thought that something may be wrong with your baby is likely to cause you a lot of worry and the seven to ten days it takes to get a definite answer from diagnostic testing can be an excruciating wait.

If the results of diagnostic testing confirm that your baby does have a chromosomal abnormality, your doctor will advise you on your options. There are varying degrees of abnormality, and your doctor and a counsellor will provide you with all the available information about the nature and consequences of the abnormality to help you make a decision that's right for you and your baby.

In Australia, approximately one in five women who conceive with IVF undergoes diagnostic testing, compared to fewer than one in ten among pregnant women in general. One explanation for this is that women who conceive with the help of IVF are usually older and so are at higher risk of having babies with chromosomal abnormalities.

Having more than one baby

The number of couples who have a multiple birth after IVF treatment has been steadily decreasing over the last few years, mainly because more and more women are having only one embryo transferred. But twins are still more common among IVF parents: In 2007, about 10 per cent of IVF parents had twins compared with a rate of 1.7 per cent for parents in general.

Even if the pregnancy goes well, carrying twins is hard work and takes its toll on your physical and emotional health. As a result, if you're having twins, you're likely to spend a lot of time being monitored during your pregnancy. You're also more likely to need bed rest during pregnancy, to deliver prematurely and to have babies that weigh less than if you had only one baby on board.

Facing complications

Don't worry yourself silly expecting complications to happen during your pregnancy: Although complications do occur occasionally, they certainly aren't the norm. However, forewarned is forearmed and in Chapter 10 I discuss the risks of pregnancy complications with IVF. It's important that you know these risks, so that any problems can be dealt with promptly.

With careful monitoring and prompt action, most complications can be dealt with successfully and mother and baby are fine.

As your pregnant body changes, you'll feel increasingly tired, bulky and uncomfortable. Some women complain about this, especially towards the end of their pregnancy, but IVF mums seem to take these changes in their stride. I think it can be hard to voice negative feelings when you've conceived through IVF — you really want your baby and you feel so lucky that IVF has worked for you. But you deserve as much sympathy as other pregnant women, so don't hold back!

Thinking About Your Baby

As they approach the birth, most pregnant women become more and more emotionally attached to their unborn baby and spend increasing amounts of time thinking about their baby. While pregnant women in general form an emotional attachment to their baby that increases substantially when they can feel the baby moving inside them, IVF mothers form a very strong and protective bond with their baby from the very beginning of their pregnancy and spend a lot of time thinking about their baby right from the start. So, if you've been hoping for a baby for a long time, you'll probably spend a lot of your pregnancy thinking about your baby.

Don't forget to leave some emotional space for your partner — you'll need your partner's full support and involvement after the baby is born! The partner sometimes feels a bit left out when attention is totally focused on the pregnant belly, so try to include your partner in your excitement and anticipation.

Imagining a real baby

Life with your real baby may be quite different to life with the baby of your dreams. In fact, some new babies turn life into a bit of a nightmare. Newborn babies often cry a lot and can be very difficult to feed, soothe and settle, no matter how hard you try. Caring for a baby is a 24/7 job and from time to time you'll be exhausted and wonder what's hit you.

Just in case you don't get a perfect, settled and content baby who sleeps through the night, it's useful to spend some time during your pregnancy getting yourself psyched up for what it may be like to have a baby with colic who cries inconsolably and never sleeps more than a couple of hours at a time. With any luck, you'll find out that thinking about having a baby who's difficult to manage was a waste of time!

All you ever wanted but ... You're allowed to feel in two minds

The transition to parenthood is a life-changing event that takes some getting used to. Becoming a parent is a new and exciting phase in your life and brings a lot of change — some for the better and some for the worse. During your pregnancy, you have time to think about how your new baby will affect your life, and acknowledge that as well as gains you may face losses, including

✔ Time with your partner

✔ Your freedom

✔ Your income

✔ Your leisure time

✔ Your pre-pregnancy body shape

Even if you've worked hard to have a baby, you're allowed to have mixed feelings about what's to come. In many ways life will get better than ever when your baby is born, but you'll also have to give up some things that you like about your current life. Ambivalence is a *healthy* emotion during pregnancy: You're better prepared to handle the losses if you allow yourself to acknowledge them before they occur.

Getting Ready for Childbirth

As your due date approaches you'll probably be looking forward to finally meeting your baby, but you may also feel a bit nervous about what the birth will be like.

It's important to be well-informed about what happens during childbirth, but you can prepare yourself only so much. How the birth pans out is largely out of your control and if you have very firm ideas about how you want the birth to be, you may get disappointed. A bit of a 'go-with-the-flow' mentality helps you be ready for whatever comes your way. In Chapter 19, I describe the different types of birth.

Planning the birth: Have your say!

About 50 per cent of women who conceive as a result of IVF have a caesarean birth, which is about twice the rate for women in general. Some of the reasons for this high rate are

- About 70 per cent of twin pregnancies are delivered by caesarean section and since IVF mums are more likely to have twins than other mums, this adds to the high proportion of babies delivered by caesarean section after IVF.

- More caesarean sections are performed in private than public hospitals, and most IVF mums have private health insurance.

- Some opt for caesarean section perceiving it as the 'safer' option. Although good medical reasons exist for having a caesarean section, contrary to popular belief it's not always safer than having a vaginal birth.

- Women who are older than age 35 when they have their first baby are more likely to have a caesarean birth than younger women, and IVF mums are usually older and more likely to be first-time mothers than mums in general.

If you have a preference for how to manage childbirth, talk to your doctor and ask for the facts about the pros and cons of your preferred way of giving birth considering your particular circumstances. Then you can let your doctor know your preferences concerning the following:

- How you want to give birth
- What kind of pain relief you want
- Whether you'd rather not have too many people you don't know attending the birth
- Whether you want to hold your baby straight away
- Who you want to bring along to support you during the birth

Making your desires known is important, but keep in mind that your birthing wish list may have to change if you or your baby don't cope well for one reason or another as the birth progresses.

Giving up paid work

If you're in paid employment while you're pregnant, you need to make plans for when to stop working. The timing may depend on your physical health and the kind of work you do, but your personal preference is also an influence. You may prefer to keep working as long as you can because staying at home makes you worry too much about the birth. Or you may stop work early because you really enjoy spending time getting everything ready for your baby and treasure the opportunity to have long lunches with your friends and rest up before your baby is born.

If you plan to go back to work during your child's first year, try to keep the timing as open as possible because the best-laid plans sometimes don't work out. After your baby is born you may find that spending time away from your baby and leaving your baby in the care of someone else is much harder than you anticipated.

Thinking Beyond the Birth

During pregnancy the event at the forefront of your mind is The Birth, and it can be hard to think beyond that point. But when you come home with a new baby you won't have much time to do anything except care for your baby, so the more you prepare before the baby is born, the better. Even more important than organising your baby's room, clothes, nappies, pram and so on is making sure that you have plenty of volunteers ready to step up to the plate when — not *if* — you need them.

Your partner is, of course, your main source of support during the birth but you'll need your partner even more afterwards. Talk to your partner about how you think you can work together to share the work of caring for your baby and running your household.

If it's practically possible, try to ensure that both of you can be home the first few weeks after your baby is born so that you can get to know your new family member together.

Caring for a new baby is tough work and even if you've waited for a long time and feel ecstatic about becoming a new parent, you'll need a break from time to time. Accept any offers of help — and get them in writing! Ask people close to you if they're willing to help out if you need them after your baby is born (they won't say no). The more people you have in your pool of helpers, the less work each of them has to take on.

If you're having twins, you'll need a small army of helpers after the birth, so start conscripting early!

Chapter 19

Welcoming Your Baby to the World

*Y*ou've been waiting for your baby's birth for a long, long time. When it finally arrives, depending on how events unfold, your experience of the birth itself can be more or less positive than you expected but, no matter what, you'll be thrilled to have your baby in your arms at the end of it. After the initial excitement of meeting your new little family member, you may start to wonder where the manual is on how to care for your bundle of joy. With a new baby, you're on a steep learning curve, but the nurses and doctors in the hospital do their best to have you up to speed with the work of new parenthood before you take your baby home.

In this chapter, I talk you through the birthing process and preparing to care for your new baby during your stay in hospital after the birth.

Arriving at 'D' for 'Delivery' Day

Whether you have a vaginal birth or a caesarean section, giving birth is very definitely a life-changing event! Unless you plan in advance to have a caesarean section, you have no way of knowing what the birth is going to be like. Afterwards you may feel that it was better — or worse — than you expected, or perhaps just like you thought it would be. No matter how your baby is born, your reward at the end of the birthing process is to hold your baby in your arms.

In this section, I explain the different types of birth, including emergencies and ones with medical issues, and talk about how you may feel during and after the birth.

Types of birth

No doubt you've had your birthing plans in place for a long time, but remember that babies have a habit of doing things their way and may completely ignore your wishes. No matter what your plans, your baby will come into the world in one of these ways:

- **Spontaneous labour:** Your waters break or you start having regular contractions, so you head off to hospital and some hours later (hopefully not too many) your baby is born.

- **Spontaneous and augmented labour:** You start having contractions and take yourself to hospital, but progress is slow or your doctor has reason to want to speed things up, so your doctor ruptures your membranes (unless your waters have already broken) and uses drugs to make the contractions more effective.

- **Induced labour:** Your doctor has reason to believe that your baby is better off out than in. You plan to have a vaginal birth, so rather than waiting for labour to start spontaneously, you book into hospital to have your labour induced with drugs and your membranes ruptured.

- **Elective caesarean section:** For any number of reasons, your doctor recommends that you have a caesarean section rather than a vaginal birth. Surgery is scheduled a week or two before your due date, and you're admitted to hospital and have your baby in the operating theatre.

- **Emergency caesarean section:** You and your doctor agree that you'll have a vaginal birth, but things don't go according to plan and your doctor resorts to plan B: a caesarean section. The decision to deliver the baby as soon as possible may be made before you start labour (for example, if the baby isn't growing as expected) or during labour if signs indicate that your baby needs to be delivered fast.

Having a birthing experience that isn't quite what you expected

Several years ago some colleagues and I undertook a study of women's experiences post-IVF (see Chapter 18). About one-third of the IVF mums in our study weren't so thrilled with their childbirth experience — but were very happy with the baby, of course! These were predominantly the women who had a caesarean delivery, as shown in Table 19-1. Some possible explanations why these women felt less satisfied include

✔ When you have trouble conceiving and need IVF to have a baby, you may want to at least be able to have a 'natural' birth. If that doesn't happen, you may feel cheated and disappointed with the way things turn out.

✔ Apart from agreeing to have the caesarean section itself, you don't have much say about what happens during the birth: You have to leave that to the experts.

✔ The ultimate reward for giving birth is to hold your baby in your arms straight away, but this isn't always possible when you have a caesarean delivery, which can be upsetting.

✔ When you have a caesarean delivery you have to put up with the post-operative pain, which probably somewhat taints your experience of the birth.

Table 19-1	IVF Mums' Satisfaction with Childbirth	
	Agreed with statement	
	Vaginal birth	**Caesarean delivery**
I had an active say about what happened during the birth.	95%	66%
I feel pleased with the birth experience.	83%	55%
I feel disappointed with the birth experience.	9%	31%
I was able to hold the baby straight away.	96%	73%
I had severe pain after the birth.	17%	32%

Some women blame themselves if they can't give birth the way nature intended. Don't give yourself a hard time about needing a caesarean section: It's not your fault and doesn't mean that you'll be less of a mother.

IVF mums and childbirth

As part of our study, my colleagues and I examined how IVF mums regard their childbirth experience and stay in hospital afterwards.

Facts and figures

About half the mums in our study had a vaginal birth, one-quarter had an elective caesarean and one-quarter had an emergency caesarean. Almost all of them said that they felt very well supported during the birth, the care they received was very kind and understanding, and they had an active say about what happened during the birth.

We compared the women who took part in our study with all Australian women who gave birth in the same year and found some interesting differences. For example, IVF mothers were

- On average five years older when they gave birth (35 years versus 30 years)

- More likely to be first-time mothers (70 per cent versus 42 per cent) and to have twins (18 per cent versus 1.6 per cent)

- More likely to give birth in a private hospital (87 per cent versus 37 per cent)

- Twice as likely to have an elective caesarean (26 per cent versus 13 per cent) or an emergency caesarean (25 per cent versus 12 per cent)

- Twice as likely to give birth prematurely (before 37 weeks) (14 per cent versus 8 per cent) and to have a baby weighing less than 2,550 grams (15 per cent versus 7 per cent)

Views about the birth experience

Giving birth is a special moment in any woman's life, but for women who have IVF treatment childbirth is also the end of a long and testing journey. Here are some recollections of the birth experiences of the IVF mums in our study:

- 'The birth was a wonderful experience, just the way I'd hoped it would be. I was so proud of myself and the way I was able to handle the pain and I remember thinking soon after Charlie was born that I could do this again tomorrow.'

- 'Because my baby showed signs of distress during labour I had an emergency caesarean under general anaesthesia. I had real trouble bonding with her for the first week and I was very disappointed that I didn't experience her being born.'

- 'I felt cheated by having a caesarean but very happy it all went well and that my baby is healthy.'

- 'I was very pleased with the birth and the care I received and my husband and I were over the moon when we heard our baby's first cry.'

Holding your baby — at last

Being able to see, hold and touch your baby is the greatest gift after nine months of waiting — not counting the time you waited before you conceived! Together you and your partner will remember and savour this moment forever.

If you plan to breastfeed and are feeling well enough, offer your baby the breast when you first get to hold her to see whether she wants to suckle. The sooner you start to practise breastfeeding, the quicker you'll both get the hang of it.

Coping when your baby needs special care

If your baby is born prematurely or has trouble breathing after being born, you may not get the chance to hold him straight away. Instead, you may see him whisked away to intensive care or a special-care nursery. Being separated from your baby is extremely distressing, and the joy you expected to feel may be replaced with tears and worry about his wellbeing.

The hospital staff usually makes sure that you get to see and hold your baby as soon as possible, even if only for a short cuddle. After they have assessed your baby's condition, they keep you informed about his progress and encourage you to be with him as much as possible.

If your baby has to stay in hospital after you're discharged, you may decide to make daily trips to the hospital to be with him. The combination of trying to recover from the birth (especially after a caesarean section), worrying about your baby, travelling to hospital and expressing milk is exhausting for mothers and emotionally very draining.

Whether you stay in hospital with your baby or travel from home every day to see your baby, try to arrange for your partner or a trusted friend or family member to be with you when you spend time with your baby. Nurses sometimes don't have time to give you much-needed support because they're busy looking after babies.

Babies have an amazing capacity to recover from a rough start in life and the specialised care that's available for newborns in Australia is exceptional, so chances are your baby will soon get better and come home so that you can get on with the rest of your life as a family.

Taking A Crash Course in Baby Care

No matter how many books about caring for babies you read, when you actually have to do it you may be surprised how unprepared you feel. When you're in hospital recovering after giving birth, plenty of experts are around you, so soak up as much good advice as you can while you're there. But most importantly, trust yourself — you'll be the expert on your own baby in no time.

Understanding that baby care doesn't always come naturally!

Baby care is an acquired skill, not something you know instinctively. Managing nappy changes and feeding, bathing and dressing your baby take practice — and you'll often wish you had three hands! Similarly, it takes time to get to know your baby and discover what she needs, and when. As you and your baby get to know each other, baby care does gradually get easier.

If you and your partner start practising baby care together while you're still in hospital, you'll both feel more confident by the time you take your baby home.

Just because you've worked long and hard to have your baby doesn't mean that caring for a newborn is any easier for you than for other new parents. In fact, in some ways it may be harder for you, because you and others around you may expect you to slip right into baby care without any problems since you finally have the baby you've wanted for so long.

Feeding: Breast is best, but ...

No doubt about it: Breast milk is the best form of nutrition for babies. But sometimes breastfeeding proves extraordinarily difficult or mothers don't feel able to do it — for example, if your baby is very sick, premature or can't suck, or if you have a health problem, you may not be able to establish breastfeeding.

Even if you can't supply all the milk your baby needs, anything is better than nothing. Whatever amount of breast milk you can provide will have plenty of goodness to help your baby grow and protect his health. If you can't provide enough for him, he can be topped up with formula.

Too many opinions

We gave the IVF mums in our study free reign to comment on anything they liked or disliked about their stay in hospital after childbirth, and the breastfeeding advice they received topped the list of negative comments by far. The two main reasons why the women were unhappy were the lack of consistency in the advice and being discharged from hospital before breastfeeding was established, as these comments show:

✔ I never had the same nurse help me with breastfeeding and every new nurse had her own techniques and ideas about how I should do it, so I was left even more confused than I was to start with.

✔ All the different opinions about breastfeeding confused me and affected my confidence in feeding for the first few weeks.

✔ I was sent home just as the milk was coming in so I didn't really have a chance to understand how to feed properly before I left the hospital.

✔ My milk didn't come in for another couple of days and that brought on major feeding problems which could have been rectified if I was still in hospital.

Although nearly all the IVF mums in our study provided some breast milk to their baby while they were in hospital, either by breastfeeding or by expressing, they didn't always find this easy. More than two-thirds needed a lot of help and advice about feeding, with first-time mothers, mothers of twins and those who had a caesarean delivery needing the most help. However, less than half of them felt that the help and advice they received was clear and worked well; in fact, many thought that the advice was confusing and didn't work.

So treat breastfeeding advice for what it is: A well-meant suggestion for how to breastfeed that works for some. But if the advice doesn't work for you, ditch it and try another piece of advice.

 Several studies have shown that breastfeeding is harder to establish after a caesarean delivery than a vaginal birth. This is partly because mums are often separated from their baby after a caesarean section and don't get to put their baby to the breast within the first hour after birth.

Finding out what works for you

When you have a new baby, everyone wants to give you their opinion about what's best for baby — whether you ask for their advice or not! The staff in the postnatal ward tell you as much as they can about the tricks of the trade during the short time you're in hospital, and after you go home your visitors all give you their two bob's worth about how to feed, burp and settle your baby. All this can make you feel as though you know nothing and your self-confidence can take a turn for the worse.

Growing a confident parental identity takes time, and when you've undergone lengthy IVF treatment, it may take a bit longer because you may have lost some of your self-confidence in the process (see Chapter 11). Don't give yourself a hard time if you find baby care challenging at first — because it really is.

By all means listen to people's advice, but keep in mind that every parent–baby relationship is unique and what works for one person may not work for you. You'll figure out what works for you and your baby by trial and error, and as you get more used to caring for your baby, you'll feel more confident.

Coping with more than one baby

If caring for one baby is tough, caring for two is extremely demanding. Twins are often born earlier and smaller than singletons and so are more likely to spend time in a special-care nursery. Smaller babies are more difficult to feed, and getting breastfeeding going with two tiny babies is definitely a challenge. Twenty-four hours isn't enough time to get through the daily work of caring for two tiny newborns and the thought of handling all this work when you leave hospital can be daunting.

Don't even try to manage caring for twins on your own; the job often requires more than both parents. Take up all offers of practical help you receive and if you don't get any offers, pay for help — even if you have to beg, steal or borrow to do so!

Making the Most of Your Hospital Stay

You'll probably have just a few days in hospital to recover after the birth, get feeding going and practise your baby-care routine, so make the most of this time. If you're in a private hospital, you may get a bit longer, and if you have a caesarean you'll definitely get some extra time to heal.

Resting while you can!

After giving birth you'll no doubt want some well-earned rest, but resting in hospital is easier said than done. Between meals being served, nurses checking on you, cleaners tidying up and your baby needing your attention, you often have precious little time for rest. If you have your own room, ask not to be disturbed if you want to rest; if you're sharing a room, pull the curtains around your bed and hope that people get the message.

Ask the nurses to look after your baby in the nursery so that you can get at least one night's good sleep before you go home. When you're rested, you have more energy to handle the demands of baby care.

Keeping visitors at bay

The phones will be ringing hot between your friends and family and soon they'll all know that your baby has arrived. Just like you, they've waited a long time to see this baby, so now they want to meet her pronto. Being showered with attention, flowers and presents after giving birth is wonderful, but you may find entertaining people exhausting when you and your partner are trying to get to know your new baby.

Apart from those closest to you, ask people who want to visit you in hospital to wait until you've been home for a while.

Getting a dose of the baby blues

The first couple of days after giving birth you'll probably be on a high and feel on top of the world. Then you wake up one morning and feel miserable, teary, irritable, confused and anxious for no good reason and wonder what's hit you. Most likely you've got the dreaded 'baby blues', which many new mothers get during the first week after giving birth. Don't worry about it — the 'baby blues' is short-lived and likely to pass after a few days. If it doesn't, let the nurses and doctors know so that they can provide the care you need to get back to your old self again.

When you have a baby after IVF treatment, people expect you to be blissfully happy every moment of the day — you've tried so hard and now you finally have a baby, so why wouldn't you be? But the 'baby blues' doesn't discriminate; you can get it no matter how you conceive. Just because you have the temporary blues though, doesn't mean that you're not happy and grateful that you've had a baby.

Feeling ready to take your baby home

After your short stay in hospital it's time to gather your belongings, take your baby home and embark on a new phase in your life. You may suddenly wonder whether you're ready for this challenge, but there's no going back. Many new parents feel quite anxious about taking their baby home from hospital. It's perfectly normal to feel worried about looking after a newborn when you've never done it before. But you can rest assured that no one will do a better job of caring for your baby than you and your partner.

Initially, IVF parents may worry more about baby care than new parents in general. This is probably because infertility and IVF treatment can rock your beliefs about your ability to look after your baby and keep your baby safe. But, of course, you're as competent as anyone else and over time you get back your trust in yourself and feel more confident about caring for your baby.

Chapter 20

Coming Home With Your New Baby

Finally, you're home with your new baby — and after just a few days in hospital, you're supposed to know how to look after her! It can be scary to realise that your baby depends solely on you and your partner, especially if this is your first baby.

Parenting is a tough gig that doesn't come with a job description. It takes time to get to know your baby and to figure out her likes and dislikes and how to make her content. And you'll find plenty to worry about: Is she putting on enough weight? Is she developing normally? Why doesn't she sleep? She cries a lot — is something wrong? All new parents worry about something, but on top of all you've been through with IVF, your worries about your baby's wellbeing can be overwhelming.

And if you don't feel enormously happy, you may wonder what's wrong with you. After all, you wanted a baby and now you have one, so why don't you feel cheerful?

In this chapter, I talk about why the first three months with a new baby are usually the hardest and give you some strategies for managing the mammoth task of caring for a newborn.

Busting Some Motherhood Myths

The birth of a baby is usually a joyful event and after you give birth to a healthy baby (especially post-IVF) you're expected to be extremely happy. But being happy about having a healthy baby doesn't make caring for him any easier. The ideas that women just *know* how to look after a baby, that motherhood is *the* most rewarding job a woman can ever do and that being a stay-at-home mum is *easy* are myths about mothering — or fathering, if dad's the primary carer — that I hereby declare *busted*.

- ✔ **Mothering isn't instinctive — even if you really wanted a baby.** You're not born with special genes for parenting — the only thing you know by instinct is that a new baby needs to be fed, cared for and protected. But how do you do this? People may presume that because you're an IVF mum you know what to do, since you've been looking forward to mothering for such a long time. But new IVF mums are as much novices to the job of mothering as other new mums, and it's normal to feel uncertain, hesitant, insecure and unconfident when you're new in a job.

- ✔ **Mothering isn't always what it's cracked up to be.** If you have high expectations of life with a new baby, the first few months can come as a rude shock. While your body is still recovering from pregnancy and the birth, you need to juggle feeding and settling the baby, washing, shopping (and that baby capsule is a monster to carry), cooking, cleaning ... the list goes on. At the end of the day you just want some sleep, but that's when the night shift starts! As much as you love your baby, the work of mothering isn't always fun-filled and pleasurable — in fact, at times it can be downright boring and exhausting.

- ✔ **Mothering needs a well-oiled team.** In most families the mother takes on the role of carer when a baby is born, but whether mum or dad is the stay-at-home parent, caring for a newborn is more than a full-time job, so extra helpers are required. You need time out now and then to clear your head, read the paper, go for a walk or have a nap. If your partner isn't available to give you a break, ask a friend or relative to look after baby while you look after your mental health.

In the paid workforce, occupational health and safety laws govern how many hours you can work without a break, how many hours off you need between shifts to allow for sleep and how often you need a meal break. If these laws were applied to stay-at-home parents, they'd all be working illegally!

Having So Much to Worry About

As a new parent, you may find yourself worrying about your baby's wellbeing: How do you know that she's had enough milk? Is she too cold or too warm? Is she getting a cold? Much of this worry stems from being new in the job and not having any experience to fall back on. After a few months when you know your baby better, you start to feel more confident in your parenting role.

Gaining maternal confidence

As part of the study my colleagues and I carried out about mothering post-IVF (see Chapter 18), we were interested to know whether we could predict which women may struggle to feel confident in their new mothering roles. We found that women who check one or more of the following statements have lower maternal confidence:

✔ Did you experience a lot of difficulty trying to conceive (for example, you were infertile for a very long time, experienced pregnancy loss and had several failed IVF cycles)?

✔ Were you dissatisfied with the care you received during childbirth?

✔ Were you anxious about caring for your baby when you left hospital after the birth?

✔ Do you have a sensitive and timid personality?

✔ Do you have an unsettled baby who is difficult to manage?

This all makes sense: Your maternal confidence takes a beating if you've been through hell and back to have your baby, you didn't feel very well looked after during the birth, you were worried about taking your baby home from hospital, you're somewhat sensitive and a bit shy, and/or your baby cries a lot and is difficult to feed and settle. It's not terribly surprising that after such experiences your maternal confidence is diminished.

More than half the IVF mums admitted to being anxious about taking their babies home from hospital. When we asked them about their confidence three months later, we found that more than half were very confident about caring for their babies and the rest — mostly first-time mums — were still a bit worried. So, even after three months' practice, you may still feel a bit tentative about baby care.

Feeling out of your depth . . .

As a competent adult who managed a demanding job, travelled the world and successfully negotiated plenty of life challenges, you may be totally surprised that a tiny baby can make you feel so out of your depth. Many new parents feel this way, but the feeling can hit even harder when you've had IVF. After you've experienced a lot of trouble having a baby, your confidence in yourself can take a dive, and this dip can cause you to doubt your ability to keep your precious baby alive.

Maternal and paternal confidence grows over time and little by little you'll worry less and enjoy your new baby more.

. . . and out of control

If you're like most people, you plan ahead and set yourself small goals to achieve every few days or so. And if you've reached your mid-thirties or later without children, you'll be used to managing your time so that you accomplish what you set out to do. So why do you now have a sinking feeling of being out of control? Because life with a new baby is surprisingly busy and quite unpredictable — just as you think your baby is getting into a regular pattern, he decides to change his routine, and the time you set aside to achieve something simply vanishes into thin air.

Try these tips to regain some control:

- ✔ Avoid putting unnecessary pressure on yourself by making too many plans in too short a period of time.

- ✔ Delete anything that's not essential from your to-do list. That way, you can enjoy anything extra that you do achieve on a 'good' day, but won't be frustrated if your baby's schedule stops you from even leaving the house on a 'bad' day.

Wondering whether you're producing enough milk

One of the many things that new mothers worry about is whether they have enough breast milk for their baby to thrive. If your baby is putting on weight every week and your maternal and child health nurse is happy with her progress, you should have no need to worry.

Food for thought

We asked the IVF mums in our study how they were feeding their babies and found that:

- Almost all started breastfeeding their babies in hospital (89 per cent)

- Compared with other mums, at three months fewer of the IVF mums were either fully breastfeeding (45 per cent versus 62 per cent) or partly breastfeeding (64 per cent versus 72 per cent)

- Over half the IVF mums continued to breastfeed their baby for more than six months (54 per cent)

- Compared with other mums, the IVF mums were more likely to breastfeed their baby beyond one year (27 per cent versus 15 per cent)

Based on these figures and comments that the women shared with us, most IVF mums hope to breastfeed their babies and do indeed start.

- If they have problems in the first couple of months or they're unsure about their milk supply, they either stop breastfeeding altogether or give their babies both breast milk and formula.

- If it's smooth sailing from the beginning and they have no worries about their milk supply, they find breastfeeding very satisfying and enjoyable and breastfeed their babies for a long time.

If you're not sure whether you're producing enough milk or you have trouble breastfeeding your baby, a lactation consultant can come to your rescue. To find a consultant in your area:

- Check out your local *Yellow Pages* under 'Lactation consultants'.

- Visit the website of the Australian Lactation Consultants' Association (www.alca.asn.au) and click on Community and then Find a Lactation Consultant.

Mother Nature is clever because the more your baby suckles, the more milk you produce. If you're keen to breastfeed your baby but concerned about whether you have enough milk, the best way to increase your milk supply is to let your baby suckle more frequently for a few days.

If you plan to breastfeed your baby and try very hard but just can't manage, you may feel disappointed and frustrated. But please don't feel guilty about it: If breastfeeding becomes a nightmare, revert to plan B — formula.

Letting sleeping babies lie

Sometimes you worry about your baby when he's asleep: Is he really breathing? So rather than having a well-earned break while he sleeps, you get all worked up about whether he's alive. You may even wake him up just to be sure he's okay!

Sudden infant death syndrome (SIDS) is every new parent's worst nightmare, but research shows that you can almost eliminate the risk of SIDS by following a few simple rules:

- ✔ Avoid sleeping baby in your bed for his first year.
- ✔ Keep all soft toys and pillows away from baby's face.
- ✔ Place baby on his back to sleep.

Stick to these rules and get peace of mind while your baby sleeps.

At the SIDS website (www.sidsandkids.org) you can find everything you need to know about how to provide a safe sleeping environment for your baby.

Caring for Baby

During the long and winding journey to becoming a parent, you build a picture in your mind of the baby you hope to have, and of course she's wonderful in every way! Your real baby may or may not be like the baby you imagined. If she is you're very lucky, but chances are she isn't quite as easy to care for as you expected.

Getting to know your baby

Every baby is unique with a distinct personality. There are no 'good' or 'bad' babies, but some babies are easier to care for than others. Very early on you get an idea about your baby's temperament: How she responds in different situations, how regular or unpredictable she is, how easy or difficult she is to settle, and how placid or energetic she is. This is the first step in getting to know your baby and can help you to work out how to best care for her.

If your baby is nothing like your imagined baby, her temperament can take some getting used to. Give yourself time to get to know your baby and to figure out what works for her.

Researchers at the University of Melbourne have put together a fantastic and very useful interactive website for new parents, called What Were We Thinking! (www.whatwerewethinking.org.au). The website has a great section on getting to know your baby: Click on the Your Baby is Unique tab in the For Parents section and then follow the worksheet instructions.

Surviving the first three months

The transition to parenthood is one of the most challenging times in your adult life. Life as you knew it is gone forever and at first you may have trouble grasping how your new life will shape up — it all just feels so chaotic. As with any major change, it takes time to get used to.

Most parents agree that the first three months with a new baby are the toughest. During this time everything revolves around the baby and you have very little time or energy for anything else. But there's light at the end of the tunnel: By about three months of age most babies settle into some sort of routine and your life starts to feel more predictable.

If your baby has a cold or is cutting a tooth, his routine can get messed up and you have to work at getting it back again when he feels better.

A very rewarding milestone in the first three months is your baby's first smile, which usually happens at about four to six weeks. Suddenly, you get positive feedback for all your efforts and feel all warm and fuzzy inside!

Crying is part of the deal, but it's hard to take

The amount of time your new baby spends crying tends to increase in the first few weeks after her birth and usually peaks at around six weeks. The sound of a crying baby is very stressful and you do anything you can to sooth her. Some babies are easy to calm, but others are very difficult. When your attempts to comfort your baby are unsuccessful, you can lose confidence and feel at a loss about what to do.

If your baby has been fed, has a clean nappy and isn't sick but still cries inconsolably and doesn't respond to anything you do to distract her, she may simply be overtired and need sleep. So, rather than distraction, your baby may need to be settled to sleep — which can be easier said than done!

Home alone

The loneliness that many new mums feel is captured in these comments by the IVF mums who took part in our study:

✔ 'I didn't enjoy the first four weeks after bringing the baby home from hospital. Sleep deprivation and monotony of baby's sleep routine and the fact that since he fed every 3 hours regardless of whether it was night or day there was no difference between my night or day … I remember thinking "Oh my God, is this what the rest of my life is going to be like?" It was all a complete shock and totally overwhelming to me not having any friends with babies, to tell me what a nightmare the first few weeks are, and the acquaintances I did know never said a word — I'm sure there is a conspiracy of silence among mothers!'

✔ 'The job is a lot harder and more tiring than I expected. I get bored, but in between it all I love my beautiful boy dearly.'

✔ 'We tried for nearly five years to have our baby, so I suppose in some ways I expected the excitement of friends and families in the first weeks of his life to continue. But of course life goes on and everyone goes back to work and it's just me and the baby home all day.'

✔ 'I feel trapped in the nicest possible way.'

The What Were We Thinking! website (www.whatwerewethinking.org.au) has a very useful worksheet to help you understand and manage your baby's crying and to recognise signs of tiredness.

Feeding can be tricky

Whether you breastfeed or bottle-feed your baby, feeding can be difficult and problems are common with newborns. Almost half of the IVF mums in our study reported having feeding problems such as not producing enough breast milk, producing too much milk and the baby refusing to take the breast or bottle.

Both you and baby are beginners at breast/bottle feeding and you need time to learn the ins and outs of the feeding routine. Don't despair if you have some teething problems at first — feeding gets easier over time.

Feeling lonely

After you bring your baby home you have plenty of well-wishers wanting to visit to see your little miracle. Although you may find entertaining exhausting in the midst of getting to know your baby, showing off your baby and receiving plenty of admiration is exciting. But soon everyone goes back to doing their own thing and then it's just you and baby.

The task of caring for your new baby fills your days (and nights!), but after the novelty wears off the humdrum of the never-ending cycle of feeding, changing and settling your baby and managing the household can become dreary. Unless you have friends who're also home alone with babies who you can spend some time with, you may find life at home with a tiny baby quite isolating and lonely.

No matter how much you love your baby and want to be with him every minute of the day, being without grown-up company day after day can be very lonesome. Try taking a daily outing, such as walking to the park to talk to some other mums with kids, to ease your sense of isolation.

See the section 'Finding Help and Support' later in the chapter for some ideas on getting out and meeting others.

Getting Into the Feed-Play-Sleep Routine

A well-tested method to get your baby into a settled pattern is the feed-play-sleep routine. If possible, you and your partner should take time to learn this routine and use it for your baby, because life takes a turn for the better when you have a well-rested baby.

During the day, this routine is as follows:

- **Feeding:** Rested babies suck well, so the routine begins with baby feeding when she wakes up. You'll find feeding a rested baby is much quicker and easier than feeding a tired baby. Table 20-1 shows how many feeds babies need in the first few months of life.

- **Time for play:** Even newborn babies need 'play' time. Your baby learns a lot about the world around her just from lying on a blanket on the floor for a little while, and her kicking and stretching help her physical development. The older she is, the longer she can stay awake to play and look around.

✔ **And so to bed:** Babies need a lot of sleep. If your baby sleeps less than 16 hours per day in the first few months, she probably isn't getting enough sleep. Table 20-1 shows how much sleep babies need in the first few months of life.

Your baby does a lot of growing and developing while she sleeps and when she's rested she cries less, is easier to feed and learns more during 'play' time than when she's tired.

Getting your baby to sleep, however, can be tricky: Try not to fall into 'bad' habits like rocking her to sleep or holding her in your arms until she's asleep — she'll only wake up as soon as you put her into her bed! Instead, your baby needs to self-settle, but getting her to do so is probably the most difficult part of establishing the routine. You need to leave her to cry until she calms down and falls asleep — but it can be heart-wrenching to hear your baby cry and not pick her up. However, after she learns to settle herself, she'll be a much happier baby.

At night-time, omit the 'play' part of the routine.

Table 20-1	A Guide to Feeding and Sleeping	
Baby's age (weeks)	*Number of feeds in 24 hours*	*Total sleep required (hours)*
0–8	6–8	16
8–12	6	15.5
12–16	5–6	15
16–24	5	14.5

Source: www.whatwerewethinking.org.au.

Settling into the feed-play-sleep routine can take a few weeks, so you and your partner need to be persistent and support each other through the process. If you're really having trouble settling your baby to sleep and it's getting you down, see the section 'Graduating from sleep school' later in the chapter.

The What Were We Thinking! website (www.whatwerewethinking.org.au) has an excellent section on what babies need, how you get the feed-play-sleep routine going and why the routine works. It also tells you how to recognise the signs that your baby is tired and provides practical advice about how to settle your baby, including how to wrap her to help her sleep.

Hard yakka

Some IVF mums from our study told us honestly how they felt about the work of mothering:

- ✔ 'I have this 24/7 job with no off-time and I do find it much more exhausting than expected. And then I feel guilty as I feel I should be more appreciative that at least I have been blessed with a child.'

- ✔ 'Looking after a baby is very tiring and there have been many days when you think you would prefer to be at work as it was easier. I think getting over the first 6–8 weeks is the biggest challenge. I also struggle with the guilt of how you should feel given the time and effort it has taken to have a baby.'

- ✔ 'Life in general is great. Looking after the baby is a lot harder and more time-consuming than I expected. The tiredness is difficult to manage at times.'

Caring For Baby Around the Clock

As a stay-at-home parent with a new baby, you're on call 24/7. Most parents get through the newborn period feeling slightly dazed — partly because the workload comes as a bit of a shock and partly because they don't get enough sleep — but they're generally happy and content in their parenting role. However, some new parents become very worn down, struggle to get through the day and don't get much enjoyment out of caring for their baby.

Never-ending invisible work

The work of motherhood/fatherhood is endless, but unlike paid work where you have set tasks to accomplish and can measure what you've achieved in a day, parenting work is largely invisible. And sometimes, although you slave away all day, you don't have much to show for your work at day's end. In fact, the dishes may still be piled up on the kitchen sink because you've spent all day trying to settle a colicky baby.

Most new parents enjoy caring for their babies but are unprepared for how demanding the work is, whether they've had IVF or not. But IVF parents don't always feel free to complain about the workload and, if they do, they often feel guilty. In addition, IVF parents may get less support than other parents from family and friends because IVF parents may feel that they should be able to manage the workload since they have a baby at last and so don't want to complain about the amount of work involved.

Parenting is a tough job: Let those around you know if you need a hand — they're sure to lend it.

Feeling down in the dumps

As a new mother, having 'bad' days when you feel frustrated, lonely and exhausted is perfectly normal. But if you feel sad day in, day out and don't find any joy in caring for your baby, you may be suffering from postnatal depression (PND). PND is a depressive illness that occurs in about 10 per cent of new mothers, and it can be very debilitating.

PND doesn't discriminate: Don't think that you can't get PND because you've had an IVF baby. Our study of IVF mums showed that PND is just as common among IVF mums as among other mums.

Warning signs of PND include

- ✔ You feel low and tearful most of the day.
- ✔ You don't enjoy your baby — or anything else.
- ✔ Your appetite changes and you have no energy.
- ✔ You have trouble getting to sleep, although you're really tired.
- ✔ You feel irritable.
- ✔ You don't feel good about yourself; in fact, you feel pretty worthless.
- ✔ You have episodes of terrifying anxiety.
- ✔ You may have thoughts of harming yourself.

Make sure that you get professional help if you feel depressed. Talk to your maternal and child health nurse or your family doctor if you think you have PND.

The organisation beyondblue is a government initiative to increase awareness about depression and improve the lives of those who suffer from depression. The organisation's website (www.beyondblue.org.au) provides in-depth information about PND and ways to manage it.

Sharing the load

The most important key to getting through the first few months with a new baby is to have adequate help and support. If you don't have to care for baby on your own and feel appreciated and supported, the work of parenting is for the most part enjoyable and gratifying.

Sharing the workload with your partner makes the experience of parenthood so much more rewarding for both of you. If your partner works outside the home, he or she can't put the same hours into baby care or household chores as you do, but his or her appreciation for the hard yards that you put in and participation in helping with the daily baby routine and other jobs go a long way to sharing the load. And hands-on parents who actively take part in the practical work of parenting give themselves a chance to really get to know and enjoy their babies.

Wondering what happened to romance

When you're recovering after pregnancy and childbirth, breastfeeding around the clock, not getting enough sleep and always keeping an ear out for baby, having sex may be the last thing on your mind. Getting back to lovemaking after childbirth can take a long time, and your sexual relationship may be different once you do.

If your sex life stalls, you can speed up the process of getting things back on track by making time to be together without baby, and being kind and affectionate and showing that you love and care for each other.

Managing with more than one baby

At least one in ten IVF births is a twin birth. Caring for two babies rather than one is in itself a colossal task, but twins are often smaller and more vulnerable than singletons at birth, which makes the job even tougher.

Here are some other issues that parents of twins need to deal with:

- **Finding a routine that works for both babies:** Twins sometimes have similar personalities, but often they don't. So you have to figure out what works for each of them and then try to get them both into a workable routine. While the babies are still little and need frequent feeds, feeding and changing babies may be all you do all day — when you're done with one, it's time for the other!

Caring for twins

Most of the mums of twins in our study had some difficulties with feeding and settling two babies and almost half found it extremely difficult to get out, do the shopping and manage housework — hardly surprising. Here are two contrasting comments about caring for twins from the mums in our study:

✔ 'Life is different. The twins have been delightful and I'm still enjoying other people's interest in them. I love my babies — our new family. I know and have experienced how hard twins can be — both crying at once is very challenging physically and emotionally, but luckily this has only happened a few times. Twins are definitely twice as nice.'

✔ 'I have moments of feeling terribly isolated and house-bound due to the fact I think of having two babies to care for. As one may be sleeping and one can be awake, not only are there days I don't get a break from "a baby" but it makes it almost impossible to get out of the house. My short walks with them are at times my saviour.'

✔ **Handling the extra workload:** Every new parent should have helpers, but parents of twins definitely need helping hands. Practical help on a regular basis is essential, particularly for the first few months. If you don't have friends and family members who're willing to volunteer, you may need to look for paid help.

If you prefer to do the baby work yourself, your helpers can do the shopping, cooking and cleaning. But if someone offers to take over baby care from time to time, jump at the opportunity and give yourself some 'time off' — you deserve it.

Finding Help and Support

The transition to parenthood can be an unsettling time that even the most resilient people struggle to handle. Most parents experience moments when they feel ill-equipped and don't know how to manage. Thankfully, a range of services in the community can help you, so take advantage and tap into these excellent resources whenever you need them.

Hooking up to Maternal and Child Health Services

When you have a baby, you become part of an amazing local government service provided Australia-wide known as Maternal and Child Health Services. Your local Maternal and Child Health Centre is notified when your baby is born and one of the maternal and child health nurses (also known as child and family health nurses) contacts you to arrange a time to visit you at home to meet you and your baby and tell you about the services that the centre provides. Your taxes are put to good work here: the services are free. Over the next few years you'll have regular contact with this nurse or one of the other nurses at the centre. The services that the centre provides include

- Assessing your baby's health and development
- Giving you immunisation advice
- Measuring and weighing your baby regularly to make sure that he's growing as expected
- Referring you to other health-care professionals should you need it
- Running mothers' groups
- Supporting and advising you about parenting, feeding, settling and anything else you may wonder about as a new parent

Joining forces with other parents

Through the Maternal and Child Health Centre you can connect with other new parents in your area. In most places the maternal and child health nurse organises information sessions for groups of new parents. When the formal sessions come to an end, a group often continues to meet on a regular basis and for many new parents such groups are a great source of support and possibly lifelong friendships.

Playgroups are also great — contrary to popular belief, kids can start playgroup at age 0, but in the early days, playgroups are definitely for mums and dads, not for the kids! You can find your local playgroup from the Playgroup Australia website at www.playgroupaustralia.com.au.

What's great about such groups is that you can chat with other mums and dads and find you're not the only one with problems and worries. And you don't have to feel shy or embarrassed about breastfeeding and changing baby in public, as you're in a 'safe' and friendly environment.

Mothers' group connections

Many of the IVF mums in our study gave testimony to how valuable mothers' groups are and how the support of other new mums helped them. But some of the mums who were in their late thirties and early forties had trouble connecting with the women in their group because of the age difference. And mothers of twins preferred to spend time with other mothers of twins (whom they found through the Australian Multiple Birth Association), because they're more understanding of what it's like to have twins.

Trawling the Web for help

Using the Web you can access as much information as you can handle about parenting. However, not all websites are worth visiting. Try these very useful and informative websites for new parents:

- **Australian Breastfeeding Association:** www.breastfeeding.asn.au
- **Australian Multiple Birth Association:** www.amba.org.au
- **Better Health Channel:** www.betterhealth.vic.gov
- **Children, Youth and Women's Health Service:** www.cyh.com
- **HealthInsite:** www.healthinsite.gov.au
- **What Were We Thinking!:** www.whatwerewethinking.org.au

Phoning for help

Help really is just a phone call away. State health departments provide a free service whereby qualified health-care professionals, including nurses and counsellors, are available to give you advice about anything relating to parenting and your own or your baby's health. Most services are available for the cost of a local call.

- **Australian Capital Territory:** Tresillian 24-hour Parent Help Line 1800 637 357
- **New South Wales:** Tresillian 24-hour Parent Help Line (02) 9787 5255 (metropolitan Sydney) or 1800 637 357 (outside metropolitan Sydney); Karitane Care Line 1300 227 464; Parent Line (Catholic Care) 1300 1300 52
- **Northern Territory:** Parentline 1300 30 1300 (8 am to 10 pm, seven days a week)

- **Queensland:** Parentline 1300 30 1300 (8 am to 10 pm, seven days a week)

- **South Australia:** 24-hour Parenting Helpline 1300 364 100

- **Tasmania:** 24-hour Parenting Line 1300 808 178

- **Victoria:** Parentline 13 22 89 (8 am to midnight weekdays and 10 am to 10 pm weekends); 24-hour Maternal and Child Health Line 13 22 29

- **Western Australia:** 24-hour Parenting WA Line (08) 6279 1200 (metropolitan Perth) or 1800 654 432 (outside metropolitan Perth)

Graduating from sleep school

In some areas you can access hands-on practical advice about baby feeding, settling and sleeping by being referred to one of the existing private or public day-stay or residential mother–baby programs. These programs help you work on solutions to your baby-care problems.

- **Day-stay programs:** You and your baby spend the day with other mums and a team of health-care professionals who offer education about baby care, individualised practical help, and advice and strategies on how to deal with the particular difficulties you're experiencing.

- **Residential mother–baby programs:** If your baby is really unsettled, suffers from colic or reflux and cries a lot and you're at the end of your tether, you can be admitted to a residential mother–baby program for a few days. These programs give you a chance to rest and get on top of your problems with the baby.

  An experienced multidisciplinary team of health-care professionals including specialist nurses, a lactation consultant, clinical psychologist and paediatrician assess your health and needs and those of your baby and put together an individualised management plan for your family. During your stay you participate in group sessions where you learn how to manage feeding, settling and sleeping difficulties and you also receive supported individualised care.

  To help parents work as a team, most programs also offer sessions for dads to get skilled up on parenting and settling techniques.

Your maternal and child health nurse or your family doctor can tell you what programs are available in your area and arrange a referral for you to attend.

In our study about mothering after IVF we discovered that many IVF mums use mother–baby programs — by three months, 40 per cent had used one program or another; most attended day-stay programs but 8 per cent were admitted to a residential program. And by 18 months 17 per cent had been admitted to residential mother–baby programs, compared with a rate of 5 per cent for new mums in general in Victoria, where we conducted our study.

Some of the many reasons why IVF mums may struggle with baby care and face the kind of difficulties that mother–baby programs can help with include

- ✔ IVF mums are older and are more likely to be first-time mums, have a caesarean section and a multiple birth.

- ✔ IVF babies are born slightly earlier and generally weigh less so can be a bit trickier to care for at first.

- ✔ Your infertility and IVF experiences can dint your maternal confidence and this can cause you to

    • Feel intense anxiety about your baby's welfare

    • Fret whether you have enough breast milk for your baby

    • Worry about how you're going to be able to keep your baby alive

- ✔ Your concern about whether your baby is okay may mean that you check on her a lot and pick her up as soon as she makes a noise. She may then get used to being carried around in your arms and have trouble self-settling and sleeping on her own.

- ✔ The idealised mental picture of motherhood and your baby you developed during your long wait for your baby can leave you unprepared for the tough reality of baby care — especially if your baby is difficult to soothe and settle, which is true of many babies.

- ✔ You (and others around you) may expect that, now you have the baby you've always wanted, you'll find looking after her a breeze and enjoy every moment of it. With such expectations asking for help can be difficult, so sometimes IVF mums get less support than other mums, although they need it just as much.

If you're wondering whether what you're doing for your baby is good enough, rest assured — no one could care for your baby better than you do. But being a new parent is emotionally and physically exhausting, so don't hesitate to ask for help and support — you need it just as much as other parents.

PERSONAL STORY

Sleeping like a log

Here's how one IVF mum explains the positive influence her stint in a residential mother–baby program had on her family:

'We were totally sleep deprived for eight months. I felt I had no control over my life and was quite depressed and teary on my own. Johnny rarely slept during the day and constantly wanted to be held, making my days very long and tiring with no relief at night.

'After waiting six weeks for an appointment I went to a settling program. There we went through some heartbreak letting him cry himself to sleep, but also learning all the sleep signs in him that we had missed and following a feed-play-sleep routine so that he didn't need to be fed to go to sleep.

'Johnny took to sleep like a duck to water, doing three day sleeps of 1.5–2 hours and 14 hours overnight. It changed all our lives for the better.'

Chapter 21

Living and Loving Life with Your New Family Member

As baby settles into a routine you find that you have a bit more energy and time on your hands, and can start enjoying outings with your baby and spending time with other parents and their babies. And now and then someone else may even look after your baby, giving you the chance to enjoy some independent leisure time — a real novelty!

Some time in baby's first year you may also need to think about rejoining the paid workforce or you may toy with the idea of having another baby. Both major undertakings require careful consideration, dedication from both partners to share the extra work and planning to carry out.

In this chapter, I talk about life after the newborn period and give you an idea of what life may be like as your baby grows.

Feeling Better Three Months On

For the first three months after your baby's born, you and baby spend time getting to know each other and you may not be totally confident in your role as a parent. But a few months down the track when you know your baby better, have a handle on what makes her happy and settled and colic is a thing of the past, you start to feel more confident about what you're doing and find you're back in something resembling control again. A daily routine emerges that makes life more predictable and allows you to fit more into your day than feeding, changing and settling your baby. And your baby may even sleep through the night — a real breakthrough for parents and baby.

I've heard this time described as 'coming out of the fog', 'feeling human again' and 'getting back into life' — the message being that there's light at the end of the tunnel of caring for a newborn.

Sleeping through the night — sometimes!

Babies vary a lot regarding when they start to sleep through the night and even when they do start, they can easily go back to night-time waking during their first two years. In a large Australian study of more than 3,000 children's sleep patterns, researchers found that

- ✔ At age three months about 70 per cent sleep through the night *occasionally*.
- ✔ Among babies who start to sleep through the night, many relapse into waking at night during their first year.
- ✔ Frequent night-time waking is common until babies are 12 months old, and one in eight babies wakes three or more times every night.
- ✔ Nearly one-third of parents report significant problems with their baby's sleep behaviour.
- ✔ Regular night-time waking becomes much less common by age two.

Babies who sleep through the night often go back to waking at night when they're teething or have a cold, nappy rash or something else that disturbs them.

From the IVF mums in our study (see Chapter 18) we found that

- ✔ At three months one in four babies was waking more than three times per night.
- ✔ At eighteen months one in five babies was still waking more than three times per night.

So, if your baby sleeps through the night regularly, consider yourself lucky — and if he doesn't, you're not alone.

Not all roses

When the babies of the IVF mums in our study reached 18 months old, we asked the mums to answer a number of questions about their overall experience of motherhood to date. The results showed that many were more satisfied with their lives as mothers than most other mums, and most found motherhood very enjoyable and rewarding. However, some of the mums were still struggling with their feelings, as these examples show:

✔ 'I think it's important that women who become pregnant after assisted conception (especially those with multiples) understand that once they are a mother, they are entitled to feel like any other mother. By this I mean that they are allowed to admit it's hard and not all roses. There is often an attitude that because this pregnancy is everything you ever hoped for that you should just be grateful and not get upset, tired etc. I myself struggled with guilt. This put extreme pressure on me and it wasn't until I admitted it was hard that I felt the pressure release.'

✔ 'Being a first-time mum I had absolutely no idea how time-consuming and at times difficult having a baby would be. I really felt a terrible failure and felt terrible when I had thoughts of "Why did I have a baby? I want my old life back" when I had so wanted a baby and tried for so long.'

For some useful tips to help you to get your baby to settle himself back to sleep after he wakes up, check out the What Were We Thinking! website (www.whatwerewethinking.org.au).

If you're having problems getting your baby to sleep and are feeling frustrated and anxious, you may benefit from a stint on a mother–baby program: Refer to Chapter 20 for more details on such programs.

Enjoying parenting

Your attachment to and love for your baby keep growing as your baby grows and increasingly your baby really feels like she's *your* baby. And as she develops you get more and more in return for your efforts — she smiles, laughs, looks for you and becomes ever-more responsive.

Don't feel guilty if you don't find motherhood/fatherhood totally gratifying and pleasurable all the time. Caring for a baby can be extremely demanding, particularly if your baby is unsettled and cries a lot.

Enjoying time with others

As your baby gets older he's awake more during the day and you may want to take him on outings. You'll find a whole world of baby-centred activities out there that you and your baby can benefit from and enjoy.

Most stay-at-home parents like spending time with other parents of young children and find their parents' group a very valuable source of company and support. With a shared interest in the nitty-gritty of teething, nappy brands and baby food, you can all give and receive advice and information and enjoy the company of others who understand what being a stay-at-home parent is all about. And as the children get older, they have fun playing with each other.

Your local Maternal and Child Health Centre can put you in touch with a parents' group to suit you: Refer to Chapter 20 for more information.

In addition to parents' groups, you can try some of these activities with your baby:

- Baby gym
- Baby massage
- Baby swimming lessons
- Library story time sessions
- Music activities
- Playgroups
- Play centres

Check out your local council's website to find out what's on in your area, or ask your maternal and child health nurse. Or you may prefer to take your baby for walks, spend time in the local park or meet a friend for coffee.

Having time to yourself

If you know someone who's willing to be your stand-in for a few hours during the day, you may appreciate having a bit of time to yourself. Having the chance to recharge your batteries every now and then by doing something that you enjoy makes the time you spend with your baby even more pleasurable.

Taking the rough with the smooth

You may find some downsides of being an IVF parent. One is that your friends may be a few steps ahead of you: You're still at home with a new baby while they're sending their kids off to school. Because a lot of parents' daily activities are tied in with the life stages of their children, you may no longer see so much of your 'old' friends when you become a new parent.

Another slight drawback, related to being an 'older' parent, is that your own and your partner's parents may be less able to help you because they're too old. They may even be in poor health and need your help at times when you need a helping hand. Several of the IVF mums in our study mentioned missing the help of grandparents and coping with the additional responsibility of caring for frail parents and parents-in-law.

Rejoining the Workforce

No matter how much you enjoy being a stay-at-home parent, your circumstances may force you to consider returning to paid work while your baby is still young. Or you may want to go back to work after some time at home.

Be aware that your plans to return to work may change after you've spent some time at home with your baby. Returning to paid work when your baby was six months old may have seemed like a good plan when you were expecting, but after you have your baby, you may not be ready to be separated from him so soon and leave him in someone else's care while you work. Unless finances dictate otherwise, you're allowed to change your mind, but if you plan to go back to your old job, you need to inform your employer if you decide to extend your leave.

Know your rights:

✔ If you worked continuously for your employer for 12 months or more before you had your baby, you have a legal right to 12 months unpaid leave and to have your old job back within that year if you decide to return to work, as long as you give your employer four weeks written notice about when you want to resume work.

✔ If you want to stay at home for longer before returning to your old job, or want to return to your old job but work fewer hours, you'll have to negotiate with your employer.

The Rudd government has promised to introduce paid maternity leave as of January 2011 — it's about time Australia caught up with the rest of the world on this!

If you have a choice about when to return to paid work, deciding the right time to do so can be surprisingly difficult. And if you decide to look for a new job, you have several things to consider:

- ✔ Deciding how many hours per week you want to work
- ✔ Finding a job that allows you to work the hours you want to work
- ✔ Finding suitable childcare
- ✔ Managing breastfeeding if your baby is still being breastfed

Returning to your old job removes the need to find a new job, but you still need to find suitable childcare and manage the breastfeeding routine if your baby is breastfed. And if you're working full-time, you may need to find someone to help with your household responsibilities.

If you're keen to continue breastfeeding your baby when you return to work, depending on the kind of work you do you can either:

- ✔ Express milk during the day and freeze it when you get home, so your baby can have breast milk from a bottle when you're not at home
- ✔ Replace daytime breastfeeds with formula or solids but continue morning and evening breastfeeds at home

Finding childcare

One of the main obstacles to returning to paid work is the scarcity of suitable childcare, because even if you're prepared to leave your baby in someone else's care, childcare can be hard to come by. Several childcare alternatives are available, depending on your budget and personal preferences:

- ✔ **Paying a family member or nanny to look after your baby in your own home:** The upside to this option is flexibility, but the downside is the high cost of paying a nanny — or finding a relative willing and able to look after your little one.
- ✔ **Placing your baby in family day care:** The upside to this alternative includes flexibility and having your baby in a family environment; the downside includes the limited places available. To find a family day care provider in your area, check out the Family Day Care Australia website at www.familydaycare.com.au or contact your local council.

✔ **Sending your baby to a crèche or day care centre:** The upside to this choice includes that most centres operate all year around, apart from a short break over Christmas and New Year; the downside includes the difficulty securing a place. To find out what childcare centres operate in your area, contact your local council. ·

✔ **Using your employer's day care facility if one is available:** The upside to this alternative is that you're physically close to your baby and may be able to see and perhaps breastfeed him during the day; the downside is that so few workplaces provide childcare.

Getting the support you need

A key to being able to combine baby care, paid employment and running a household without going under is having the necessary practical support. When you take on paid work, your partner may need to make some adjustments to his or her work schedule, so that household responsibilities are still accomplished.

Finding the right balance

We quizzed the IVF mums in our study about how they combined motherhood and paid employment and discovered the following:

✔ When their babies were three months old, 23 per cent of the mums were doing some paid work and five dads were acting as stay-at-home parents while their partners were in full-time employment.

✔ When their babies were eight months old, 46 per cent of the mums were in paid employment, and this increased to 60 per cent when the babies were 18 months old.

✔ Most mums worked part-time, but 12 per cent worked more than 40 hours per week.

✔ Most mums felt that the time they spent at work was about right and were happy to combine baby care with employment, but 26 per cent felt that their working hours were too long.

✔ More than two-thirds of the mums who weren't working when their baby was 18 months old weren't planning to return to paid work in the foreseeable future.

The message seems to be that if you can find the right balance and work the hours that suit your needs, combining parenting and paid employment can be rewarding and stimulating.

You may need to find alternative practical support if your partner works long hours and can't share the workload at home. Paying someone to help regularly with cleaning, cooking, ironing and/or gardening can be money well spent.

Trying For a Sibling

Unless you've decided that your family is complete, you may start thinking about another baby at some point. Because IVF couples in general are older than other couples when they have their first baby, they tend to get the urge for another baby sooner rather than later.

Starting IVF again

If you know that you have to undergo IVF to conceive again, you need to bite the bullet and get on with it. Ask your family doctor for a new referral to your infertility clinic and then make an appointment to see the IVF doctor. Your IVF doctor will arrange for you to have any tests that need updating, then you can see the IVF nurse and get your instructions to start another IVF cycle (refer to Chapter 5 for a refresher on what the cycle entails). Having been there and done that already, you won't find the IVF experience as daunting as when you started your first cycle.

Going back to IVF for baby number two can be easier in some ways because you know the ropes and what to expect. But the disappointment you feel if the treatment doesn't work isn't easier to take the second time around. And don't listen to people who say you should be grateful that you've been successful already: If you want another baby, you're entitled to feel sad if the treatment doesn't work.

Using frozen embryos

Having frozen embryos in storage gives you a chance to have another baby without needing to go through all the steps involved in an IVF cycle. You still need to ask your family doctor for a new referral to your IVF clinic and to see your IVF doctor before having the frozen embryo transferred, but the process is pretty straightforward. Depending how regular your menstrual cycle is, the IVF nurse will advise you what you need to do to get ready for embryo transfer. (I explain the steps in frozen embryo transfer in Chapter 5.)

Adding to the family?

When their babies were 18 months old we asked the IVF mums in our study if they were hoping to have more children and here's what they said:

- 50 per cent were hoping to have more children

- 20 per cent hadn't decided whether to have more children

- 25 per cent didn't want more children

- 5 per cent couldn't have more children

- 8 per cent had experienced pregnancy loss since their baby was born

- 20 per cent were pregnant or already had another baby — most of these women had actually conceived spontaneously but some had been through IVF again

Fluking it by getting pregnant without help

Some couples unexpectedly conceive another baby spontaneously even though they needed IVF to have their first baby. This can come as a bit of a shock, particularly if you get pregnant within a few months of giving birth. After the long hard road to having your first child, you may have trouble comprehending how you can possibly conceive without any help from the lab.

Unless you know that you definitely *can't* conceive without IVF, there's always a chance that the stars will align and you'll conceive spontaneously. So, if you don't want a surprise pregnancy, talk to your doctor about contraception. But if you want more children and don't mind when, who knows — you may just get lucky!

Part VI
The Part of Tens

Glenn Lumsden

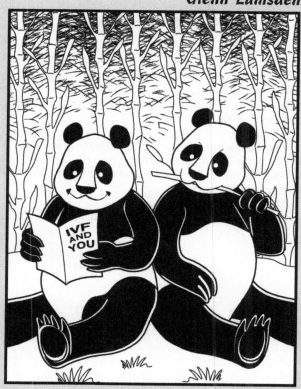

The bear facts

In this part . . .

*I*f you're extremely busy and don't have time to read a bunch of full chapters, want the short and sweet about having IVF treatment and prefer to deal with things when they happen rather than anticipating them, this part is perfect for you.

In this part, I outline ten very important points to help you keep sane during your IVF treatment and ten tips to make the transition to parenthood after IVF as smooth and enjoyable as possible.

Chapter 22

Ten Tips for Surviving IVF

In This Chapter

▶ Keeping yourself informed

▶ Being there for your partner

▶ Enrolling supporters

*1*VF is a very high-tech way of getting pregnant and you have to get your head around all sorts of medical jargon and complicated instructions, not to mention putting up with the inconvenience of numerous clinic visits and all that poking, probing and prodding of your body along the way. But that's the easy part: The trickiest aspect of IVF for any couple is hanging on to each other and your sanity during the ups and downs of treatment.

In this chapter, I give you ten survival tips to help you through IVF.

Gathering Information

Before undergoing IVF treatment you need to gather as much information as you can, so that you have an idea of what to expect and can make informed decisions about your treatment options. Most importantly, knowing how IVF can affect your emotional health and finding out about strategies to help you cope with treatment make you better equipped for the IVF journey. Refer to Chapters 9 and 11 for more information about the emotional aspects of IVF.

If you've already read this book — particularly Part II — you can actually tick this first tip off your list!

Working Together

Infertility is a couple problem, irrespective of who has the 'faulty part', and you and your partner need to work together to try to overcome your problem. Tune into each other and make sure that you're both fully committed to IVF before you start treatment, because you need each other's love, care, support and nurturing throughout the IVF process and beyond, whether treatment works for you or not. I talk more about supporting your partner in Chapter 9.

Helping Each Other

In Chapter 5 where I explain the IVF process, I describe IVF as a set of hurdles that you have to jump over: If you don't clear a hurdle, you have to start again. A lot's at stake when you have IVF, and when treatment doesn't go to plan, it's very disappointing. You invest so much physical and emotional energy, time and money in the process that any setback can make you lose heart and feel low and discouraged. Refer to Chapter 9 for some tips on managing the highs and lows during your IVF journey.

As you go through the trials and tribulations of IVF treatment, don't forget to keep an eye out for your partner and be there for each other if things don't go to plan.

Avoiding the Guilt Trip

When you first find out that you're infertile, you and your partner probably ask 'Why us?' There's no good answer to this question — it's just a fact that about 15 per cent of couples who try to have a baby discover that they have a fertility problem. You're not infertile because you've done something wrong — you're just unlucky. So don't blame yourself or your partner, because it's not your fault you're having difficulties. Instead of looking for someone (or something) to blame, looking for solutions like IVF is much more productive.

Setting Limits

You may hit the IVF jackpot and fall pregnant straight away, or you may need a few 'goes' to get pregnant — and sometimes IVF just doesn't work at all, no matter how hard you try. When a cycle is unsuccessful, your IVF doctor talks you through the details of your treatment and estimates your chances of treatment working if you try again. You then have to decide whether you're prepared to have another go. You need to be in the driver's seat and make an informed decision about how many times you'll try, so set a limit for how many cycles you'll have, even if you later decide to go beyond that limit if you're not quite ready to give up your baby dreams.

In Chapter 8, I give you some advice on how to calculate the chances of IVF working for you and to set some realistic goals for your treatment.

Escaping Together

IVF can become all-consuming, so be mindful that it doesn't take over your life completely. While you're undergoing treatment you're naturally preoccupied with the treatment and may find thinking about anything else very difficult. You also have a schedule to stick to, which can restrict your freedom to do things like travelling and going on holiday.

Make a conscious effort to fit some fun into the mix and escape the grind of treatment when you can, even if you only manage a short weekend away with your partner.

Talking to Someone Else

As much as you want to be there for your partner, from time to time you may both be feeling under the pump and unable to lend support to each other. Close friends, parents and siblings can be wonderful sources of encouragement and support and are likely to be more than happy to be your sounding board if you let them. Talking to someone who isn't directly involved in your treatment can give you a new perspective and help you get back on an even keel.

Finding Virtual Support

You'll find an array of websites dedicated to infertility and IVF treatment, and many have facilities for people to chat and share their experiences. From the comfort of your home you can connect with people who really understand what you're going through because they've had similar experiences to yours — even though you don't know them or live on the same continent. If you like the idea of talking about your feelings and sharing your experiences of infertility and IVF while remaining anonymous, the internet is perfect for you.

If you enter 'infertility support' into your favourite search engine, you're likely to get more than ten million results! You can narrow your search down by adding 'Australia', but you'll still get more than two million results. So you may need to spend a bit of time figuring out which sites you find useful. In Appendix C, I list some Australian online support groups.

Turning to a Counsellor

IVF clinics in Australia and New Zealand are required to make counselling services available to couples who attend their programs. Infertility counsellors are experts on the emotional aspects of infertility and infertility treatment and can help couples to make informed decisions about their treatment options. You can benefit from a counsellor's experience and expertise at any stage of your treatment. For example, you may want to talk to a counsellor if you:

✔ Experience pregnancy loss

✔ Have difficulty deciding whether to continue with or stop treatment

✔ Receive bad news about your treatment and need to talk to someone who understands IVF about what this means for your future chances of having a baby with IVF

✔ Struggle in your relationship or have trouble communicating with your partner

✔ Suddenly feel overwhelmed by everything and unable to manage the strain of the infertility and the rigours of treatment

Knowing When to Stop Treatment

If you have multiple treatment cycles without success, how do you get off the treadmill? Some couples feel that they *can't* stop treatment because that spells the end of their baby dreams. And sometimes one partner wants to keep going with treatment while the other wants to move on.

There's no right or wrong time to stop treatment, but you and your partner need to think carefully at what point you'll bring your efforts to have a baby to a close and move on with your lives. Talking to your IVF doctor or a counsellor can be helpful in reaching your decision about when to stop IVF.

In Chapter 12, I give you some strategies for coping when you conclude that enough is enough and decide to move on with your life.

Although the outcome of IVF is out of your control, you still have control over how many treatment cycles you have and can decide to stop when you've had enough.

Chapter 23

Ten Tips for New IVF Parents

Congratulations: You've cleared all the IVF hurdles and you're pregnant! As you close the door on your IVF treatment and enter the world of antenatal care, you can start to count the days until you finally meet your baby. The transition to parenthood is an amazing and joyous period that starts in pregnancy. But becoming a parent for the first time can be pretty daunting and unsettling, even if you've endured a long hard road to get there.

One of the difficulties that some IVF parents face is that their expectations of themselves as parents, their baby and life with a newborn are somewhat romantic and idealised, and don't match the real-life experience of caring for a little one. Added to this, friends and family expect IVF parents to be blissfully happy and find parenting a breeze.

The truth is, kissing goodbye to your life as you knew it and getting on with your new role as a parent with responsibility for the care and survival of a newborn baby is a mammoth task for all new parents, IVF parents included.

In this chapter, I give you ten tips for new IVF parents that pretty much all boil down to a single message: Feeling out of your depth, hesitant, doubtful and uncertain in your new role as a parent is normal, and you don't need to feel guilty if you don't enjoy every moment of it — even if you *are* lucky enough to have a baby with IVF.

Preparing for Pregnancy Probing and Prodding

As an IVF mum, expect many check-ups, tests and examinations during your pregnancy. There are many reasons for this scrutiny:

- ✔ Doctors and midwives sometimes feel extra-protective of women who conceive with IVF.
- ✔ IVF mums are generally older than other mums and therefore have a slightly higher risk of pregnancy complications.
- ✔ Most IVF mums are first-time mothers.
- ✔ Twins are more common after IVF than with spontaneous conception.

If you want to enjoy the natural process of pregnancy, you may not appreciate the high-level surveillance you get when you're pregnant. But if you worry about whether your baby is doing okay, you may be reassured by your frequent antenatal check-ups.

I talk more about pregnancy tests, check-ups and screening in Chapter 18.

Some women feel exceptionally well and positively glow during pregnancy, whereas others suffer a lot of physical discomfort or have to be hospitalised because of pregnancy complications. Don't feel guilty and, above all, don't blame yourself if you don't enjoy every moment of your pregnancy — such feelings don't mean that you're ungrateful.

Imagining (Real) Life with Your Baby

Most pregnant women spend time thinking about their baby and imagining their life after the baby is born. And when you're happy about being pregnant and looking forward to becoming a parent, your thoughts are predominantly positive and full of anticipation. But you need to factor in and accept the losses that inevitably come with parenthood too, such as:

- ✔ The changes to your body that happen after childbirth
- ✔ Your freedom to come and go as you please and choose what you do with your time
- ✔ Your independent leisure time — unless you consider a trip to the supermarket without the baby as leisure!

✔ Your professional identity and income — at least temporarily

✔ Your relationships with your partner and others, which may change as you shift most of your attention to the baby

Ambivalence is a normal and healthy part of pregnancy that helps you settle into your new role as a parent when your baby is born.

Handling Birthing Plan Letdowns

Childbirth is a unique experience that every pregnant woman anticipates with mixed feelings. Countering your excitement of meeting your baby for the first time is the trepidation about what the birth will actually be like.

If you're hoping to have a vaginal birth and end up having a caesarean, you may feel cheated and disappointed — after all, you needed IVF to conceive, your pregnancy was super-monitored and to top it off you end up having a caesarean delivery. You may feel overwhelmed by all the technology and resentful that nothing seems to be straightforward and 'natural'.

In Australia, more than 50 per cent of IVF mums have a caesarean section, which is twice the rate of other childbearing women (I explain why this is so in Chapter 18). Given these odds, it's a good idea to be prepared for this eventuality. And, if you're over 35 and expecting twins, you're almost guaranteed to have a caesarean birth, so you may as well make your birthing plans accordingly.

You mustn't give yourself a hard time about needing a caesarean section. You've done nothing to deserve your tough road to motherhood: It's not your fault that your way has been paved with complications and high-tech medical interventions.

Having the Confidence to Take Baby Home

After only a few days practising the art of parenting in hospital, you're expected to be responsible for caring for this tiny creature. Feeling anxious and unprepared for this enormous task is perfectly normal — especially if you've never done it before. IVF mums sometimes worry even more than other mums: It's as if the stumbling blocks on the way to parenthood diminish your maternal confidence and self-belief in your capacity to care for your baby. But, no matter how out of your depth you feel, remember that your baby is in good hands and could have no better parents than you.

Facing Life at Home with a Newborn

Bringing a new baby home can be a bit of a shock — nothing prepares you for the time and energy required keeping up with the needs of a newborn. Baby care is a skill that you learn, not one you're born with. Every newborn is different and you need time to figure out what works for your baby and what doesn't. Trusting that what you're doing is right for your baby and feeling confident in your role as a mother takes a bit longer for some IVF mums, but over time your confidence grows and you enjoy your baby more and more.

I explain how to establish a good feed-play-sleep routine for your newborn in Chapter 20.

Figuring Out the Intricacies of Baby Feeding

Even if you have every intention of breastfeeding your baby, you may have problems and find this 'natural' process harder than you thought. Unfortunately, the advice about breastfeeding you receive can be conflicting — and sometimes bad.

If you have a strong wish to breastfeed your baby, don't give up, and remember that some breast milk is better than no breast milk — your baby will benefit even if he's partially breastfed and topped up with formula. I talk more about establishing breastfeeding in Chapter 19. You can also try these resources if you're having problems:

- Day-stay programs to facilitate breastfeeding (ask your maternal and child health nurse for a referral)
- Private lactation consultants (check your local *Yellow Pages* under 'lactation consultants')
- The Australian Breastfeeding Association (visit www.breastfeeding.asn.au)
- Your maternal and child health nurse

If you really want to breastfeed your baby and try very hard but it just doesn't work, don't beat yourself up over it: Babies who're given formula thrive too, and both you and baby may feel better if feeding isn't a constant battle.

Coping with Baby Care 24/7

Baby care is relentless and many new mothers find the job much harder than they thought. Your life is dictated by your baby's needs, leaving little, if any, time for you. Until your baby is settled into a routine — and that can take many months — your day is pretty unpredictable and you usually find you achieve little apart from caring for baby and getting through (some) household chores. You may even feel a bit lonely after the rush of visitors is over. And you certainly need more sleep than you get. Considering the workload, feeling worn out is normal. But if you feel really low, irritable and worthless, have trouble enjoying your baby (or anything else), can't sleep even when your baby sleeps and your appetite changes, you may be suffering postnatal depression (PND).

If you suspect that you have PND, don't suffer in silence. PND is a condition that requires professional help, so talk to your maternal and child health nurse or your family doctor as soon as possible.

Make That Two: Caring For Twins

One in ten IVF mums comes home with two newborn babies. Anyone who's cared for one baby can imagine what doubling that workload would be like (and shudder at the thought). Don't even try to manage two newborn babies on your own. Take up *all* offers of help that you get and, if that's not enough, get some paid help if you can afford it.

Sharing the Load

Whether you have one baby or two to look after, as a stay-at-home parent you need practical help, emotional support and a bit of time to yourself occasionally. The first port of call for this help is your partner. Whoever does the paid work in your family needs to be prepared to help out after work and take over some of the baby care and home duties. Working parents who take an active part in the care of their baby get doubly rewarded: Their stay-at-home partners are happy and they get to know and enjoy their babies.

Reaping the Rewards of Parenthood

If you're overwhelmed by the demands of caring for your newborn and wonder when life is going to feel 'normal' again, don't despair. After the first crazy few months of new parenthood the dust usually settles and things start to look up. You may get the odd night of decent sleep, your baby has some sort of a routine, you know what your baby wants when she 'calls', you feel confident about caring for her, and you get plenty of rewards for your efforts when your baby giggles and shows her toothless gums.

Even if your confidence about caring for your baby is a bit shaky at first, rest assured that you're not alone and very soon you'll be an expert on looking after your baby. Research shows that confidence about caring for the baby grows over time and most IVF mums and dads find parenthood enormously rewarding and fulfilling. Perhaps the long and winding IVF journey, during which you realise that you can't take parenthood for granted, makes you appreciate and value parenting even more than if you'd had a baby the quick and easy way.

Part VII
Appendixes

Glenn Lumsden

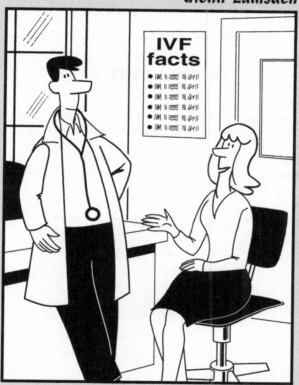

'When you said you were giving me a gift,
I didn't realise you meant a Gamete
Intrafallopian Transfer. But if it
works, it'll still be a gift.'

In this part . . .

The language of IVF is full of technical terms and acronyms and you can sometimes feel 'lost in translation'. In this part I explain terms that you'll probably come across while you're on the IVF program and point you to some websites that you may find useful on your IVF journey.

Appendix A

Abbreviations

· ·

AID	artificial insemination donor
AIH	artificial insemination homologue
AMH	anti-müllerian hormone
ANZICA	Australian and New Zealand Infertility Counsellors Association
β-hCG	beta human chorionic gonadotrophin
BMI	body mass index
CC	clomiphene citrate
cd	cycle day
CVS	chorionic villus sampling
D&C	dilatation and curettage
DI	donor insemination
ET	embryo transfer
EV	estradiol valerate
FET	frozen embryo transfer
FSA	Fertility Society of Australia
FSH	follicle-stimulating hormone
GIFT	gamete intrafallopian transfer
GnRH	gonadotrophin-releasing hormone
hCG	human chorionic gonadotrophin
HIV	human immunodeficiency virus
HSG	hysterosalpingogram
ICSI	intracytoplasmic sperm injection
IVF	in-vitro fertilisation
IVM	in-vitro maturation
LH	luteinising hormone
MESA	microsurgical epididymal sperm aspiration

NHMRC	National Health and Medical Research Council
NPSU	National Perinatal Statistics Unit
OHSS	ovarian hyperstimulation syndrome
OI	ovulation induction
OPU	oocyte pick-up
PBS	Pharmaceutical Benefits Scheme
PCO	polycystic ovaries
PCOS	polycystic ovarian syndrome
PESA	percutaneous epididymal sperm aspiration
PGD	pre-implantation genetic diagnosis
PN	pronuclei
RANZCOG	Royal Australian and New Zealand College of Obstetricians and Gynaecologists
RTAC	Reproductive Technology Accreditation Committee
TESA	testicular sperm aspiration
TESE	testicular sperm extraction

Appendix B

What Does This Mean?
(A Glossary of Terms)

· ·

adhesions: Scar tissue that stops the fallopian tubes from moving freely.

amenorrhea: Absence of periods.

andrologist: A doctor specialising in the male reproductive organs.

aneuploiy: Having an abnormal number of chromosomes.

anovulation: When ovulation doesn't occur.

antisperm antibodies: Antibodies that 'attack' sperm and make them clump together so that they're unable to fertilise the egg. Also known as *sperm antibodies*.

artificial cycle: A cycle in which you take medication to mimic the hormones produced by your ovaries in a normal menstrual cycle, in preparation for the transfer of frozen embryos.

artificial insemination: Placing washed sperm in the uterus to help a woman to conceive.

assisted hatching: A technique whereby the embryologist makes a small hole in the zona pellucida to help the embryo hatch.

asthenospermia: Not enough sperm swimming forward.

asthenoteratospermia: Not enough sperm swimming forward and too many with abnormal shape.

azoospermia: No sperm.

beta human chorionic gonadotrophin (β-hCG): A pregnancy hormone that's measured in your blood after embryo transfer.

blastocyst: A five- to six-day old embryo.

blastocyst transfer: Transfer of embryos that have reached the blastocyst stage.

blastomeres: The individual cells in an embryo.

blighted ovum: A pregnancy without a foetus.

cervix: The neck of the womb.

chromosome: A DNA structure that contains the genes and is found in every cell of the body. Normal cells have 46 chromosomes: 23 inherited from the mother and 23 inherited from the father.

cleavage stage embryo: An embryo in its first stages of development.

clinical pregnancy: A pregnancy where clinical signs such as a gestational sack or a foetus are evident.

clomiphene citrate (CC): A drug in tablet form that stimulates follicle growth.

commissioning couple: A couple who enter an agreement with a woman to carry a pregnancy for them.

cryopreservation: Freezing.

culture medium: Fluid containing all the nutrients essential for embryo development.

cycle: The time from the start of one period to the start of the next.

cycle day (cd): Each day of the menstrual cycle; the first day of the period is cd 1.

day two to three transfer: Transfer of embryos two or three days after egg collection.

donor-conceived child: A child born as a result of egg, sperm or embryo donation.

donor conception: A pregnancy conceived using donor eggs, sperm or embryos.

donor embryos: Embryos formed from the eggs and sperm of one couple and subsequently donated to another infertile couple.

donor gametes: Donor eggs or donor sperm.

ectopic pregnancy: A pregnancy that implants and starts to grow outside the uterus, often in one of the fallopian tubes.

egg collection/retrieval/pick-up: An ultrasound-guided procedure whereby eggs are removed from the ovaries for the purpose of IVF treatment.

eggs: The female germ cells.

embryo: The developing human from the time of implantation to eight weeks' gestation.

embryo biopsy: The removal of one or two cells from an embryo to check whether the embryo is normal.

embryo cryopreservation: Embryo freezing.

embryo transfer: When embryos are placed in the uterus.

embryologists: Highly trained scientists who specialise in embryo culture.

embryonic stem cell research: Research to determine whether embryonic stem cells, which are cells that have the potential to develop into any type of cell in the body, can cure chronic illnesses.

endometriosis: A condition whereby the tissue that lines the inside of the uterus (the endometrium) finds its way to other places in the body.

endometrium: The lining of the uterus.

estradiol valerate (EV): Synthetic oestrogen in tablet form.

fallopian tubes: The two tubes that at ovulation transport eggs from the ovary to the uterus.

female factor infertility: Couple infertility due to a female problem.

fertilise: When the sperm penetrates the egg.

flare protocol: A short hormone stimulation protocol for the simultaneous growth and maturation of multiple eggs.

foetus: The developing human from eight weeks' gestation until birth.

folic acid: A B vitamin that helps develop healthy cells.

follicles: Fluid-filled sacs in the ovaries where the eggs develop and mature.

follicle-stimulating hormone (FSH): One of the hormones produced by the pituitary gland in the brain that regulates the menstrual cycle.

follicular phase: The first part of the menstrual cycle from the start of a period until ovulation.

fragmentation: Disintegration of one or more cells in an embryo.

gamete: Egg or sperm.

gamete intrafallopian transfer (GIFT): A procedure whereby eggs and sperm are placed in one of the fallopian tubes to help a woman to conceive.

gene: The basic hereditary unit made up of DNA and located in the chromosomes.

genetic condition: A health condition caused by 'faulty' genes.

gestation: Pregnancy.

gestational carrier: A woman who carries a pregnancy for another man and woman (the commissioning couple), who then raise the child. Also known as *surrogate*.

gestational surrogacy: A pregnancy carried by a woman who agrees to hand the baby to the commissioning couple after birth. Also known as *surrogacy*.

gonadotrophin-releasing hormone (GnRH): A hormone produced in a part of the brain called the hypothalamus, responsible for the release of follicle-stimulating hormone and luteinising hormone, two hormones that regulate the menstrual cycle.

hormone: A chemical released in one part of the body that affects cells in another part of the body.

human chorionic gonadotrophin (hCG): A hormone produced by a growing pregnancy that is used in IVF to mature eggs because it has the same effect as luteinising hormone, which initiates oocyte (or egg) maturation and ovulation in the menstrual cycle.

hydrosalpinx: A blocked fluid-filled fallopian tube.

hysterosalpingogram: An X-ray of the uterus and the fallopian tubes.

hysteroscopy: Examination of the inside of the uterus.

idiopathic infertility: Infertility that has no apparent cause.

incubator: A container for developing embryos in the lab where a constant temperature and oxygen concentration are maintained.

infertility: The inability to conceive after one year of unprotected intercourse.

intracytoplasmic sperm injection (ICSI): A procedure used for male factor infertility where a single sperm is injected into an egg.

in-vitro fertilisation (IVF): Literally 'fertilisation in glass'; refers to fertilisation occurring in a lab rather than in the body.

in-vitro maturation (IVM): Immature eggs maturing in the lab.

IVF counsellor: A mental health professional specialising in the psychosocial aspects of infertility and IVF treatment.

IVF doctor: A doctor specialising in infertility and IVF treatment.

IVF nurse: A nurse specialising in the treatment of infertile couples having IVF treatment.

laparoscopy: A minor surgical procedure that allows the doctor to thoroughly examine a woman's fallopian tubes and uterus.

lifestyle modification programs: Programs aimed at improving general health to increase a couple's chance of pregnancy.

long protocol: A long hormone stimulation protocol for the simultaneous growth and maturation of multiple eggs.

luteal phase: The second part of the menstrual cycle, from ovulation until the next period.

luteinising hormone (LH): One of the hormones produced by the pituitary gland in the brain that regulates the menstrual cycle; its most important job is to trigger maturation and release of the egg (ovulation).

male factor infertility: Couple infertility due to a male problem.

menarche: A young woman's first period.

menopause: The time of a woman's life when her ovaries stop producing eggs.

micromanipulator: A specialised piece of equipment with joysticks that allows embryologists to perform precision work such as ICSI and PGD under the microscope.

microsurgical epididymal sperm aspiration (MESA): Withdrawal of sperm from the top part of the testicle.

miscarriage: Pregnancy loss before 20 weeks of gestation.

oestrogen: A hormone produced in the ovaries, primarily before ovulation.

oligoasthenoteratospermia: Too few sperm, too many with abnormal shape and not enough swimming forward.

oligomenorrhea: Irregular and infrequent periods.

oligospermia: Fewer sperm than normal.

oligoteratospermia: Too few sperm and too many with abnormal shape.

oocyte: Egg.

ovarian hyperstimulation syndrome (OHSS): A potentially dangerous over-response to hormone stimulation.

ovarian reserve: The potential capacity of the ovaries to produce eggs.

ovarian stimulation protocol: A combination of drugs used to stimulate the simultaneous growth and maturation of multiple eggs.

ovaries: The part of the female reproductive organ where eggs are stored.

ovulation: The release of an egg from the ovaries.

pathologist: A doctor specialising in the analysis and measurement of components in body fluid and tissue.

percutaneous epididymal sperm aspiration (PESA): Withdrawal of sperm from the top part of the testicle.

polycystic ovarian syndrome (PCOS): A hormone imbalance that affects many bodily functions, including ovulation.

polycystic ovaries (PCO): Large numbers of small follicles in the ovaries.

pre-implantation genetic diagnosis (PGD): A technique whereby a cell is removed from an embryo to check the number of chromosomes and whether it's affected by genetic problems, so that only healthy embryos can be transferred.

premature ovarian failure: When the ovaries stop producing eggs in women under the age of 40.

primary infertility: Couples who have never conceived.

progesterone: A hormone produced in the ovaries, primarily in the second phase of the menstrual cycle after ovulation.

pronuclei (PN): Structures seen in eggs after fertilisation. If an egg has fertilised normally, two PN are seen the day after egg collection — one containing the genetic material from the egg and the other containing material from the sperm.

secondary infertility: Couples who are unable to conceive again after having one child or more.

short protocol: A short hormone stimulation protocol for the simultaneous growth and maturation of multiple eggs.

'slow freeze' method: An embryo cryopreservation technique whereby the temperature of the embryos is decreased over a period of some hours before they are placed in liquid nitrogen to avoid ice forming inside the cells.

sperm: The male germ cells.

sperm antibodies: Antibodies that 'attack' sperm and make them clump together, so that they're unable to fertilise the egg. Also known as *antisperm antibodies*.

stimulation response: The number of eggs produced in response to hormone stimulation.

success rate: The chance of having a baby with IVF.

supernumerary embryos: Embryos that a couple doesn't want or need.

surrogacy: A pregnancy carried by a woman who agrees to hand the baby to the commissioning couple after birth. Also known as *gestational surrogacy*.

surrogate: A woman who carries a pregnancy for another man and woman (the commissioning couple), who raise the child. Also known as *gestational carrier*.

teratospermia: Too many sperm with abnormal shapes.

termination: Abortion.

testicular biopsy: Removal of small pieces of tissue from the testicles.

testicular sperm aspiration (TESA): Withdrawal of sperm from the testicles.

testicular sperm extraction (TESE): Withdrawal of sperm from the testicles.

ultrasonographer: An expert at interpretation of ultrasound imaging.

ultrasound: A non-invasive method using soundwaves to produce images of organs in the body, including a growing pregnancy.

uterus: The womb where the fertilised embryo implants and grows.

vasectomy: A minor surgical procedure whereby the tubes that carry the sperm from the testicles to the penis are tied, rendering the man sterile.

vitrification: A quick cryopreservation technique whereby embryos are placed in a droplet of a particular solution and then immediately placed in a special container that's cooled by liquid nitrogen.

zona pellucida: The layer of specialised cells surrounding the egg (the 'egg shell').

Appendix C

Web Resources

The amazing World Wide Web is a great resource that you can tap into from the comfort of your own home or the local library. The only problem is finding useful and reliable information. Below I suggest some excellent websites that you may find helpful.

Breastfeeding

- **Australian Breastfeeding Association:** www.breastfeeding.asn.au
- **Australian Lactation Consultants' Association:** www.alca.asn.au

Childcare and playgroups

- **Family Day Care Australia:** www.familydaycare.com.au
- **Playgroup Australia:** www.playgroupaustralia.com.au

Infertility and postnatal emotional support

- **ACCESS, Australia's National Infertility Network:** www.access.org.au
- **Australian Infertility Support Group:** www.nor.com.au/community/aisg
- **beyondblue:** www.beyondblue.org.au
- **Donor Conception Support Group:** www.dcsg.org.au
- **FertileThoughts:** www.fertilethoughts.com
- **SANDS Australia, Stillbirth and Neonatal Death Support:** www.sands.org.au
- **The Surrogacy Center Australia:** www.surrogacyaustralia.com

Infertility causes

- ✔ **Andrology Australia:** www.andrologyaustralia.org
- ✔ **Centre for Genetics Education:** www.genetics.com.au/home.asp
- ✔ **The Jean Hailes Foundation for women's health:**
  - • **Endometriosis:** www.endometriosis.org.au
  - • **Managing PCOS:** www.managingpcos.org.au

IVF laws and regulations

- ✔ **Assisted Reproductive Technology Act (New South Wales):** www.health.nsw.gov.au/hospitals/phc/art.asp
- ✔ **Fertility Society of Australia:** www.fsa.au.com
- ✔ **National Health and Medical Research Council Ethical Guidelines:** www.nhmrc.gov.au/publications/synopses/e78syn.htm
- ✔ **Reproductive Technology Council (Western Australia):** www.rtc.org.au
- ✔ **South Australian Council on Reproductive Technology:** www.dh.sa.gov.au/reproductive-technology/default.asp
- ✔ **Victorian Assisted Reproductive Treatment Authority (formerly Infertility Treatment Authority):** www.varta.org.au

Looking after baby

- ✔ **Australian Multiple Birth Association:** www.amba.org.au
- ✔ **Better Health Channel:** www.betterhealth.vic.gov.au
- ✔ **Children, Youth and Women's Health Service (South Australia):** www.cyh.com
- ✔ **HealthInsite:** www.healthinsite.gov.au
- ✔ **Sids and Kids:** www.sidsandkids.org
- ✔ **What Were We Thinking!:** www.whatwerewethinking.org.au

Miscellaneous

- ✔ **Low Cost IVF Foundation:** www.lowcost-ivf.org
- ✔ **Medicare:** www.medicareaustralia.gov.au
- ✔ **Quitline:** www.quitnow.info.au

Index

Notes

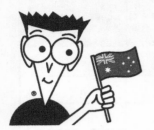

FOR DUMMIES®

Business & Investment

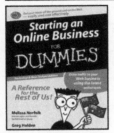

0-7314-0991-4
$39.95

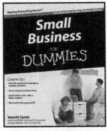

1-74216-853-1
$39.95

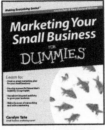

1-74216-852-3
$39.95

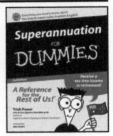

0-7314-0715-6
$39.95

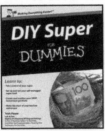

1-74216-943-0
$39.95

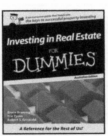

0-7314-0724-5
$39.95

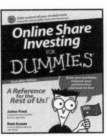

0-7314-0940-X
$39.95

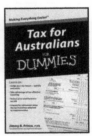

1-74216-859-0
$32.95

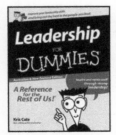

0-7314-0787-3
$39.95

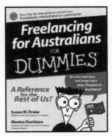

0-7314-0762-8
$39.95

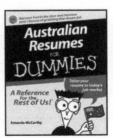

1-74031-091-8
$39.95

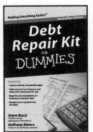

1-74216-941-4
$36.95

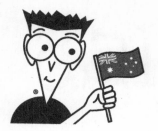

FOR DUMMIES®

Reference

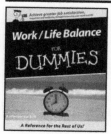

Work / Life Balance

0-7314-0723-7
$34.95

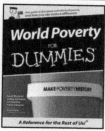

World Poverty

0-7314-0699-0
$34.95

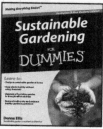

Sustainable Gardening

1-74216-945-7
$39.95

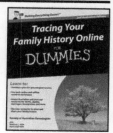

Tracing Your Family History Online

0-7314-0909-4
$39.95

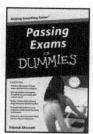

Passing Exams

1-74216-925-2
$29.95

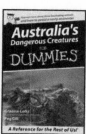

Australia's Dangerous Creatures

0-7314-0722-9
$29.95

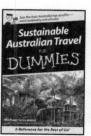

Sustainable Australian Travel

0-7314-0784-9
$34.95

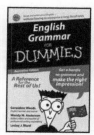

English Grammar

0-7314-0752-0
$34.95

Technology

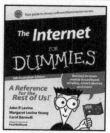

The Internet

0-7314-0985-X
$39.95

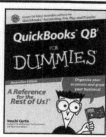

QuickBooks QB

0-7314-0761-X
$39.95

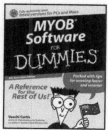

MYOB Software

0-7314-0941-8
$39.95

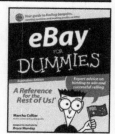

eBay

1-74031-159-0
$39.95

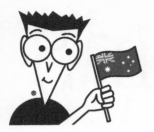

FOR DUMMIES®

Health & Fitness

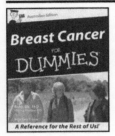

Breast Cancer

1-74031-143-4
$39.95

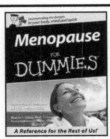

Menopause

1-74031-140-X
$39.95

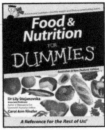

Food & Nutrition

0-7314-0596-X
$34.95

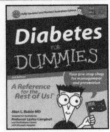

Diabetes

1-74031-094-2
$39.95

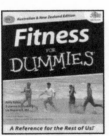

Fitness

1-74031-009-8
$39.95

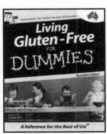

Living Gluten-Free

0-7314-0760-1
$34.95

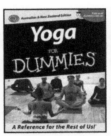

Yoga

1-74031-059-4
$39.95

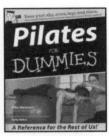

Pilates

1-74031-074-8
$39.95

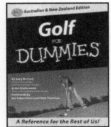

Golf

1-74031-011-X
$39.95

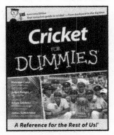

Cricket

1-74031-173-6
$39.95

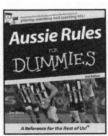

Aussie Rules

0-7314-0595-1
$34.95

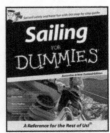

Sailing

0-7314-0644-3
$39.95

Printed in Australia
16 Mar 2016
447563